First Aid
for My Horse

First Aid for My Horse

By Anke Rüsbüldt

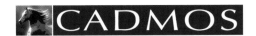

Copyright © 2005 by Cadmos Verlag, Brunsbek
Translated by Annette Brooks, BA, Dip.Trans.IoL, MIL, MITI
Project Management by the Editmaster Co, Northampton
Typesetting and Design: Ravenstein, Verden

Printed in Germany.

ISBN 3-86127-914-2

Contents

1 How to Avoid Emergencies and First Aid

First aid for horses is undoubtedly an important area of knowledge for anyone who keeps, rides or simply loves horses. First aid is always a practical skill and, accordingly, is not something which can merely be learned theoretically from a book. My intention here is to set out the most important theoretical principles of first aid in a comprehensible way, and to encourage the reader to practise the skills described. More specifically, my concern is to explain all the risks which our horses can run, as clearly as possible, so that you can take precautions and thereby avoid having to use your newly acquired first aid skills at all. Over the years, I have offered courses under the headings of "First Aid for Horses" and "How to Recognise and Avoid Risks to Horses". Only the first of these ever attracted any interest! And this despite the fact that most emergencies arise out of situations which could have been avoided, as a result

of thoughtlessness, high spirits, carelessness, laziness, meanness or plain ignorance.

The avoidance of emergency situations is thus more important and easier than first aid. However, first aid will always be needed, because accidents and mishaps will occur, even where the greatest care is taken.

Reading this book will show you how to assess situations correctly, and to react carefully and skilfully to each situation – to do what is necessary in each individual case and to leave out anything which is unnecessary. Piling in with blind enthusiasm does more harm than good. You will train yourself to remain calm and not to lose your head in situations from which you would normally rather run screaming.

Practise keeping your own and your assistants' safety in mind. You are no use to anyone if you have just been kicked into the corner. Practise describing situations – as you would do to a vet or the fire brigade, for example.

Create good conditions for you and your horse to work in, and ensure that they are maintained.

There is, of course, a great deal that you can do yourself. This is already the case, and once you have read this, you will be able to do even more, or do it better. In a real emergency, you will still always need the assistance of a vet. Your task will be to care for the patient until the vet arrives, to support the vet in his work and to provide tender loving care to the patient – not the vet.

Incidentally, a small point about vets: I myself am a female veterinary surgeon specialising in horses, and I am convinced that the difference between the sexes is of absolutely no relevance in the attribution of professional and humanitarian aptitude for this profession. For the purposes of readability, I will continue to refer to "the veterinary surgeon" as the male of the species, and this will also apply to the horse-owner, the animal practitioner and the yard-owner. Readers who are militantly minded feminists may make whatever manuscript amendments they feel appropriate.

Also, I will not distinguish patients by height or type of use. An injured pony gelding "of no value" experiences the same feelings of panic and pain as his larger friend with more competition success under his belt. The term "horse" will be the principal term of reference for all horses or ponies.

In individual cases, the distinction may be relevant in deciding what kind of future the patient will have, and whether someone is prepared to invest time and money in him. The concept of animal protection thus gives rise to the concern about whether a particular therapy is appropriate and reasonable for the horse. However, this is not a decision which you will have to make alone and, in the first instance, surely every injured horse has the right to be helped.

Problems will always arise, of course, if owners cannot or refuse to pay the costs they have incurred by calling out the "wrong" vet. Such difficulties, however, arise rarely and you will only reproach yourself, if you failed to do everything you could have done for the horse.

In the first instance, it is a question of saving life, taking away pain and minimising loss. Everything else is "only" money.

I hope that you will benefit from this book, and that your horse will never encounter a real emergency situation.

Personal qualities

Staying calm is the most important thing to do, because you will be able to get an overall perspective:
- What has happened?
- What, in the worst case scenario, is likely to happen next?
- Have any people been injured or are they in any immediate danger?
- Have any animals been injured or are they in any immediate danger?
- When did it happen?
- What can I do?

- What do I need?
- Where is the nearest telephone?

The best thing is to answer these questions while the shock is still "live". Don't panic. If you can do this, you will have met the most important personal criterion. You will be calm and collected, and you will remain master of the situation.

Be clear in advance as to what you can do. If, for example, you can't see any blood, go and find a telephone and delegate care of the patient to someone else. If you tend to stammer in stressful situations, it would be better to delegate the telephoning to someone else. If you are a small-framed woman with little body mass, let others pull ropes. If you are big and strong, don't hang back – you will be needed.

This has nothing to do with discrimination, but where there are a number of people, the results will be better if each person does what he is best able to do.

One person should telephone, one should look after the people involved, another should try to calm the horse and another should keep a lookout at the roadside in order to avoid delays in locating the accident site.

If you are alone, if possible, don't leave the horse, and don't remove any other horses. Only remove tack or similar items if you are unlikely to need them. With any luck, you will have a mobile phone with you – with a fully charged battery.

Do not put yourself in danger. The horse knows you and, of course, he never kicks. However, in an emer-gency situation, the horse may be fearful, or even panicky and in pain. His reactions will be sudden and uncontrollable. If you are injured, you will no longer be in a position to help, and any helpers will help you first. Never forget how strong a horse can be.

You will also need to be able to assess the horse's condition accurately and to prioritise your actions. This can be learned partly by reading – as you are now – partly by experience and partly by practising selected exercises. Administering first aid incorporates a number of techniques which can and need to be practised, such as bandaging or the use of the twitch. Consider organising a special first aid course with the help of your vet, a qualified equine nurse or animal practitioner.

You should wear stout, non-slip footwear and long trousers. You may also need gloves. Shorts and sandals are pretty and comfortable in summer, but impractical for doubtful situations. When you are around horses, get into the habit of wearing clothing and footwear which, if need be, will stand up to extra pressure.

What will I need?

Of course, virtually every yard has a first aid kit or cupboard. Unfortunately, most of the time, this usually consists of a collection of opened and/or empty tubes of creams, over-flowing and sticky eye lotions and a number of rags which were once bandages.

Take the time to put together a

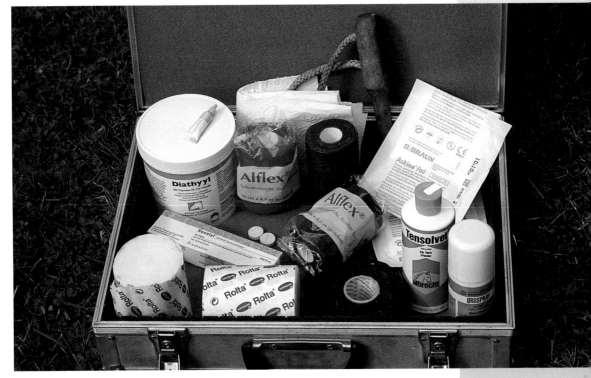

yard first aid kit on an emergency-free day, and discipline yourself to replace items immediately if you need to use them. Check the contents and the use-by dates of drugs regularly. The yard first aid kit is for everyone to use and should be accessible to everyone (not kept in a locked cupboard or at someone's house). What may also prove useful is to prepare a small first aid kit to take with you either on a hack or to a competition, so that you always have the most necessary items with you without the need to break into the main kit.

What the yard first aid kit should contain
- Sterile dressings (non-stick ones are best)
- Padding: cotton wool or gamgee, poultice (such as Animalintex)
- Self-adhesive elastic bandages (such as Flexoplast or Vetrap)
- Sticky tape
- Scissors for bandages and curved edge scissors
- Disinfectant solution (such as Pevidine)
- Wound cream for superficial abrasions
- Thermometer.

The following can also be useful:
- Stethoscope (with a little practice, you can listen to the heart and lungs yourself)
- Twitch (to be used only in extreme cases as a means of persuasion. Practise putting it on a few times. Do not practise tightening it.)

- Wire cutters (how else would you remove a leg from wire?)
- Farriery tools (shoepuller and claw hammer for removing nails)
- Clean cloths
- Clean water
- Soap
- Plastic bags
- Bran for poulticing
- Wound powder/healing gel/green oils
- Cooling gel/ice-pack
- Emergency drops (Bach flower remedies)
- Torch
- Latex gloves.

In any event, the following should always be available: good quality ropes (no quick-release fasteners), lead ropes or flat webbing straps and strong, well-fitting headcollars in good condition.

For legal reasons, and because you will not want to invest all your money in drugs, you will not be able to put together a complete drugs cabinet. It is better to buy each new drug individually, as and when you need it. Don't be fooled by offers you may receive via the Internet or junk mail from dealers offering cheap drugs. These people are only offering prescription-free drugs, which are also available to you over the counter. Everything else is illegal.

Drugs such as wormers and vaccines on offer from outside the European Union are untested. They may well also be counterfeit.

Bargains on feed supplements can be achieved if you buy them in bulk and, if possible, order direct from the manufacturer. Bandages are also cheaper if you buy them in packs, rather than singly.

Drugs which are efficient are generally prescription-only, and can be obtained from your vet or from a pharmacy.

Homoeopathic treatments should also only be used following a diagnosis, but you can certainly keep a homoeopathic preparation such as Traumeel in the form of tablets or cream. This is a complex preparation which has a positive influence on all types of cuts, bruises and similar injuries. Horses who often suffer from colic or have difficulty in passing urine can be successfully treated with Nux vomica. Discuss the use of these treatments with an animal practitioner. There is no point in collecting a whole arsenal of natural remedies, because many of the effective ones spoil easily and are sensitive to heat and light.

They are not necessary for first aid. If you subsequently decide to use supplementary medicines in order to influence the healing process, they can be obtained from your local pharmacy within 24 hours.

A dry, level and preferably well-lit area makes things a great deal easier.

A kettle will raise comfort levels and will make it easier to dissolve drugs. Electrical equipment and points should be in good condition and checked on a regular basis. A kettle which sets the yard alight is more of a hindrance than a help.

Even if horses are kept at grass, a box or separate area should be available for sick animals. If it can be positioned so that the patient can still see his field companions, so much the better. Make arrangements amongst yourselves to provide company for the patient. For instance, a second animal could be kept with the patient on box rest in rotation. Try to make such arrangements in a non-emergency situation, so that no one party is put in the position of seeking favours. General rules are there for everyone and, of course, no-one knows who may be affected next.

A supply of hay and non-palatable bedding (shavings, hemp or peat) should be kept in reserve for days on which the shops are closed.

A lightweight rug should also always be somewhere to hand.

Transport for injured horses should be available, or at least easily arranged. Here, too, agreement in advance is necessary. It doesn't matter how many trailers are standing in the car park, if they are all locked, can't be used for interpersonal reasons or are unroadworthy. A vehicle to tow and someone who is willing and able to drive are required. If your own horse is affected, you may be too nervous or upset, or you may be injured, if you and your horse were involved in the accident together. Neither is it a good idea to be towing a trailer for the first time with an injured horse. Organise contacts with a professional transporter and make a note of his mobile telephone number. Make a trip to the local veterinary clinic, so that you will know the way and what you can expect when you get there.

A telephone should be available or accessible. A note of important numbers is best kept next to the phone – in a stressful situation, you may only remember part of the number for the veterinary surgery. A note of the address and telephone number of the yard should also be kept next to the phone, so that it can be given to the vet or the fire brigade. If there is no telephone in the yard, consider buying a mobile phone which everyone can use.

For every horse, the telephone number on which the owner, sharer or another authorised person can be reached should be available. If you have to leave a message, don't leave hair-raising details, just ask the person to call back. A panicky or shaky voice asking the person called to "pick up the phone" may make it impossible for them to react calmly. The fact that someone from the yard has called is generally frightening enough. Leave your number for the call to be returned.

It is also good if information on every horse is available – date of the last tetanus jab, allergies to medicines and preferred veterinary surgeons.

In case of colic, it would be good to have previously thought about whether, in the event, the animal is to be taken to an animal clinic (and if so, which one) and also whether the animal should be operated on. More about this in the section on colic, p. 64.

In the event, you must be able to find your way to the relevant animal clinic quickly. Leave directions (most clinics will provide a map). Misplaced optimism along the lines of "Don't worry, I'll find it" could waste precious time. Let the clinic know what time you expect to arrive.

Outside help

If you are sufficiently experienced and have a basic knowledge, you will be able to treat minor injuries yourself. Normally, in situations where first aid is required, a second person will be needed.

Urgent veterinary attention will be required in the following cases:
- heavy bleeding
- the horse is unable to put any weight on one leg
- severe symptoms of colic
- severe swellings appear on the head
- there are symptoms of a blocked gullet
- the horse is cast
- there are serious wounds on the croup
- there are gaping wounds
- injuries are sited in particularly vulnerable areas
- there are complications during foaling
- the horse presents significant circulatory problems
- there are respiratory difficulties
- the horse is stumbling around or appears not to be aware of its surroundings.

You may also need to seek veterinary attention if:
- the horse's temperature is above 39°C
- there are possible symptoms of colic
- there are wounds that have stopped bleeding or if bleeding is minimal
- you are unable to assess the extent of the injury
- there are injuries to the hoof
- the horse is scouring

- the horse is coughing
- the horse has a nosebleed
- you notice something unusual.

In principle, it is better to call the vet once too often than not enough. Leaving aside the moral question of animal protection and our duty of care, the cost of the consequences of failing to take action in the initial stages usually far outweighs the cost of an unnecessary call-out.

If you need veterinary help urgently, you can call more than one vet. Once the first vet has arrived, you can cancel the others; however, you will have to reimburse each of the others who has already rushed off to help you. Please try to ensure that you initiate this type of vet-racing only in the most dire of emergencies. If the first vet you call confirms that he will be with you in twenty minutes, don't call anyone else. The only thing that matters in an emergency is that the horse receives professional help as rapidly as possible.

You will need the help of the fire brigade in the following circumstances:
- the horse has been involved in an accident in a trailer
- the horse has collapsed or has fallen into a ditch and is unable to get out by himself
- the horse is so badly cast, that he can only be freed by mechanical means.

A few skilled farmers and yard-owners will be able to do this themselves, but the fire brigade is a skilled, competent and helpful force which is available to everyone 24 hours a day.

My personal experience of the fire brigade in horse-rescue cases has always been very positive.

You should notify the police if:
- horses are wandering on the motorway or on a main road
- roads or junctions have to be closed in order to carry out a rescue operation
- a horse has strayed.

Organise yourself so that you can provide all the necessary personal details, or appoint someone to provide the police with the information they need. There is absolutely no point in yelling impatiently at an officer who is trying to do his job in the correct order. Make sure that cars belonging to helpers, the vet, onlookers and others at the scene are not in the way. The Highway Code applies, even in an emergency situation. If a horse has an accident in a trailer, try, if it is possible without further harming the horse, to move the vehicle and trailer off or to the side of the road. Never open the front ramp on the trailer.

Other riders, grooms and yard staff will, of course, offer assistance. However, someone has to take charge and ensure the safety of volunteers.

Strangers, who may not be experienced with horses, should not be directly employed in helping the horse. With a trailer accident, for example, you may have helpful drivers on your side. Explain to them when you will need their help and exactly what they should do, but never forget what a danger an injured horse can be, not only to himself, but also to those around him.

If you are extremely lucky, a qualified equine first-aider, an experienced breeder or someone with years of experience will be on hand. Listen to their advice and agree on what you are going to do. If you are the most experienced person there, make your decisions and take firm charge, in order to avoid the dangers of people just doing their own thing. Delegate tasks by speaking directly to people and give precise instructions (for example: "The gentleman in the yellow jumper – would you please come here and keep this rope taut" is better than "Could somebody please hold this?").

Damage to third parties should, if possible, be recorded immediately (photographs). This saves trouble with insurance companies later on. Make notes on the following lines, for example: a helper has been kicked; one helper's new leather jacket has been torn, the wing of a car has been dented, a borrowed trailer has unfortunately been destroyed, leather tack has had to be cut, and so on. It is far easier to remember this type of detail on the day, rather than weeks later when you are filling in an insurance claim form.

2 Assessment of the Patient

We should, of course, be in a position to distinguish between a healthy horse and a sick one. The transition can be swift, and recognition requires knowledge and practice. A horse which is cast or has been involved in an accident can be instantly classed as an emergency, but the question "Do I need a vet now or at all?" requires more accurate insight. You will also make it easier for the vet to assess the patient's condition if you can describe its symptoms accurately.

It makes good sense to be able to carry out a brief health-check on a horse by yourself. It is immensely reassuring and puts the situation into perspective. With a little discipline, the gradual onset of changes in the horse will also be detected sooner. However, please do your horse a favour and don't overestimate him. If in doubt, always call the vet.

Every patient has an age, a sex, a breed, an owner and a name. Even this basic description provides a clearer picture. The breed does not necessarily include how the animal was bred. An example of this is a pre-visit report in which I was told that "The two-year-old Appaloosa mare has colic". This description led me to expect that the horse in question was of normal size. Lola, however, was a miniature Appaloosa standing only 10.2hh, which meant that the rectal examination I had planned was technically impossible.

It can be important for a vet to have some idea of what he can expect to find, amongst other reasons, so that he can bring the right equipment.

An impacted testicle can cause a stallion to present severe colic symptoms; some drugs should not be given to pregnant mares; young animals react differently to older animals, and so on.

If the animal is known to the vet, he will be able to recall previous ill-

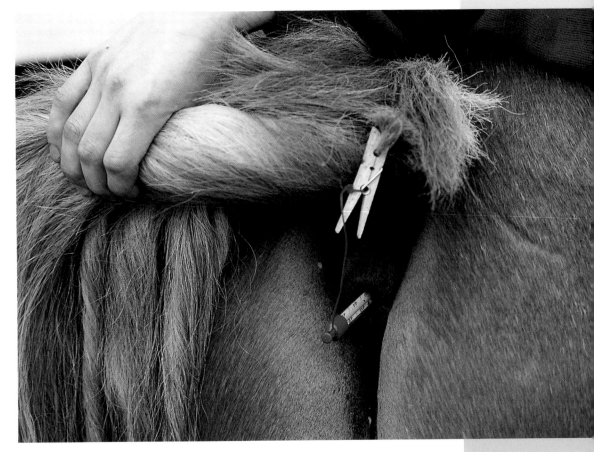

How to take a horse's temperature. The thermometer is attached to a cord tied to a peg, which can be clamped to the tail.
Photo: Dr. Ende

nesses, individual disposition or drug intolerances to mind en route.

In every case of illness, it is useful to establish basic parameters such as pulse and respiratory rate and to take the temperature.

A good pre-visit report for colic cases should also include information on whether there are any gut sounds, the severity of the symptoms, times of last feed, last work and, if possible, the last time droppings or urine were passed (when, quality and quantity). All this information will provide you and the vet with a better opportunity to assess the condition of the patient correctly.

In cases of shock or scouring, you can measure the degree of dehydration, or the capillary filling time for circulation problems yourself. How? Read on.

Where a leg has been injured, it is possible to tell by feel which structures may have been affected. The position of foreign bodies (glass shards or nails) in the feet should be ascertained as accurately as possible.

Where bleeding is heavy, it is possible to assess the amount of blood lost.

Even without carrying out specific examinations, it is possible to establish quite a lot merely by observation.

The healthy horse

A healthy horse will stand on all four legs and will be aware of and interested in his surroundings. A healthy horse will also lie down from time to time, doze standing up, or rest on alternate hind legs, but he can be brought into the state defined as healthy (woken up).

The horse behaves normally. What constitutes normal behaviour cannot be defined generally or specifically here. Abnormal behaviours are pawing the ground, rolling, looking at his stomach, running round in circles, staggering, falling down, flehmen, chewing with an empty mouth or coughing. Some healthy horses display some of these behaviours in certain situations. The better you know your horse, the easier it will be for you to distinguish between what is normal and what is not. Be on the alert for small things.

The coat is smooth and shiny and there are no signs of injury. Of course, some horses grow a shaggy coat in winter, which can get dirty, but watch out for injuries and loss of shine.

The eyes of a healthy horse are clear, the pupils wide and there is no discharge. The eyelids are free of injury.

The nostrils are dry and not flared.

The legs show no sign of injury or swelling, the hooves look uninjured from both the top and the underside.

There are no traces of faeces on the insides of the thighs, and for mares, no discharge of vaginal secretions.

The respiratory rate is around six to fourteen breaths per minute. With the horse at rest, the number of breaths can be counted by watching the movement of the flanks. A horse breathes costo-abdominally, that is, he uses both his rib-cage and his abdomen during breathing. If the horse is using more of his abdomen, and if you can see that this abdominal breathing is strained, and there is a line along the abdominal wall, this is abnormal.

The horse has a good appetite and drinks plenty.

The droppings are round and moist, with an aromatic odour.

Urine is passed easily and in a continuous stream. The urine itself is a pale yellow colour. Frothing is normal.

The visible mucous membranes are pale pink with no spots or wider areas of blood. When a horse has colic, these membranes are a yellowish, grey or blue colour. The yellowish colour also appears when liver disease is present, if the horse is starving, or in other situations in which the horse is feeding poorly. The blue colour appears when breathing is impaired or if the horse is asthmatic.

At this stage, you already know quite a lot about the horse's current state of health. Now go on and find out more.

The pulse rate should be between 28 and 40 beats per minute. You can measure the pulse rate from under the chin. The underside of the lower jaw bone has a dent in which you can feel the blood vessels. By applying light pressure, you can feel the pulse. It will be even easier if you have a stethoscope which you can call your own and have practised a bit of auscultation. Place the stethoscope behind the elbow on the left-hand side. Wait a moment for the horse to get accustomed to the feeling, then listen in and count. Very few horses will stand still for a whole minute so that either your hand or the stethoscope does not slip.

Look at your watch and count the pulse beats for 15 seconds. Then multiply the count by four. A pulse can also be found in the legs by special examination of the limbs (see p. 20).

Body temperature is between 37°C and 38°C. To measure body temperature, place a thermometer between 4 and 5cm into the anus and hold it there for three minutes before taking a reading. Digital thermometers are faster and make a beeping sound when they have finished taking the temperature. Let your horse hear the sound before you take his temperature, to avoid him taking fright at the wrong moment. If the horse is not used to having his temperature taken, ask someone to hold his head. If you don't want to hold the thermometer all the time, it can be attached to a clothes peg by a cord, and the peg fastened to the tail. Body temperature rises after work or after eating, and a measurement taken at such times will not be accurate. Every horse will also have his own individual normal temperature. The best thing to do is to take your horse's temperature morning and evening over a few days, and then you will know what is normal. If the horse's temperature is constant at 37.2°C, then he will already be ill if the temperature suddenly measures

38°C, which you would not have noticed if you had not known his individual normal temperature. Horses whose temperature is always 38°C would not be a cause for concern until their temperature reached 38.5°C. The surface temperature of the skin can and should be felt. In cases of allergies or urticaria, horses are often warmer in various places, although their rectal temperature does not rise. Where injuries involve nerve-endings, some areas of skin will be literally dripping with sweat. Increased heat in a leg or hoof will be discussed in the section on special examination of the limbs. In order to establish the condition of the circulatory system, you can measure the elasticity of the skin and measure the time it takes for the capillaries to fill. Elasticity can be measured by pinching a fold of skin at the neck. When it is released, the fold should flatten immediately and not leave any

Testing elasticity by pinching a fold of skin. Photo: Dr. Ende

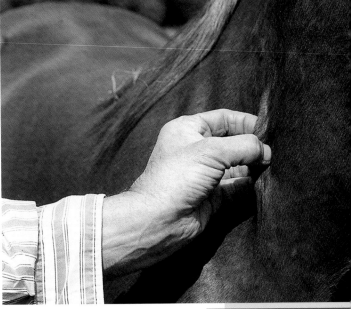

visible marks. If the fold takes a while to flatten out, it is a sign of dehydration. Capillary filling time is measured by the mucous membranes in the mouth. Pick up the top lip so that you can see the mucous membrane. Press on the membrane with one finger. As soon as you remove your finger you should be able to see a white mark, which should return to the same pinkish colour as its surrounding membrane with a maximum of two seconds.

These two parameters will tell you something about dehydration and peripheral circulation. They are important signs in cases of colic, shock, scouring and heavy bleeding.

Special examination of the limbs

The point of this exercise is simply to discover the extent of any damage. If a horse is unable to put any weight on a leg, or if it is bleeding heavily, veterinary attention should be sought as soon as possible. Injuries to the hoof will always require veterinary attention. A horse which cannot put any weight on a leg or which refuses to move should be left exactly where he is. Never try to move him, not even as far as the stable. Fractures, fissures, torn tendons or ligaments, laminitis and tying up are made worse by every step. Ideally, the vet will come to the site of the accident, otherwise – and after consultation with the vet – the injured horse should be transported.

Ascertain whether the horse can and/or is willing to move straight forward. If he absolutely refuses, this may be because of severe pain in one or more limb, or he may have tied up.

While the horse is standing, feel for increased heat in separate areas of the limbs by laying your hand flat over the area. The pulsation of the arteries to the toes can be felt at the coronary band. You will always be able to feel this, so practise! Increased pulsation is a clear and important indicator of infection below that point. It is very often the case that the rate of pulsation increases and heat in the hoof rises when the horse suddenly goes lame. The cause can be a hoof abscess (this often occurs during moulting, and lameness is high-grade and worsening), stepping on a nail, another type of hoof wall injury or laminitis. The vessels leading to the toes can also be felt under the inside of the carpal joint on the foreleg, and under the hock on the hind leg. You will, in fact, only be able to feel a pulse here if the hoof is injured or diseased. This makes practice difficult. Have a good look at the legs. Did he have that lump there yesterday? Feel any new swellings: are they hard, soft or fluctuating (this is when they feel like a water-filled balloon)? Are they getting larger? Where a fracture or fissure has occurred, swelling is generally very evident. Fracture haematomas swell as you watch them; you can clearly see them becoming thicker. Are the new swellings warm? Does it hurt if you press on them? You must be very gentle when applying any pressure to such swellings. The horse's reactions will vary greatly, depending on the degree of pain he is feeling. There are some horses who will simply remove any person who dares to add insult to injury by pressing on a point which already hurts from their field of vision, with one swift, clean movement. This can be very painful. There are also some very well-behaved horses in whom you can only see that that pressure is really rather uncomfortable just now by the expression on their faces or because they are holding their breath.

Look at the hoof wall: is it intact, underneath as well as on top? Watch out for gradual changes. In the early stages, thrush can be detected by sight and smell. Small stones should be removed from the white line area, and shod hooves should be inspected daily. It costs very little time or effort to pick out the feet every day (even if you are only lungeing today). That way, you can save your horse unnecessary bruising caused by a stone he picked up the day before yesterday. If, when you pick up a foot, you notice part of a foreign body sticking out underneath, think twice before you react instinctively and start to pull it out. If only the head of a nail is showing, then it is possible, while the nail remains in the hoof, to find out (by X-ray if need be) what it has damaged on the way in, and how deeply and in what direction it has penetrated the foot. Once it is removed, it will leave only a channel, which will rapidly swell and close. If you must pull it out, make a mental note of the entry point, depth and direction of penetration. Bandage the foot immediately (see p. 24). Don't

be too easily impressed by symptoms – look carefully. With injuries to the hoof, or so-called hoof abscesses, the infection can cause the whole leg to swell, or just the pastern, or even just the heel. The hoof itself, of course, cannot swell, but it can be the cause of swelling. A horse-owner who greets the vet with "It's the fetlock, it's really swollen" is generally surprised to see that, after a short observation, the vet removes a stone which has become wedged in the cleft of the frog. Usually, he also feels a bit silly. You can spare yourself such embarrassment!

Try to lift the leg you have decided is affected. Can the joints be moved without hurting? Can you lift the opposite leg, so that the horse has to put all his weight on the affected leg? You should only be trying to form a picture. If it doesn't work, or causes pain, stop.

Feel down the cannon bone on the leg you have lifted. Try to feel each tendon separately and follow it down the leg. Get someone to show you how to do this. It is always good to be able to feel your horse's leg for abnormalities on a day-to-day basis. If horse-owners could do this, over half of all tendon damage could be avoided. You will already have noticed structural changes, swellings (small ones, of course, otherwise prevention wouldn't be so difficult), heat or pain several days before the damage becomes visible. Examining all four legs like this every day after riding takes about three minutes (about twenty hours a year, and time is money: but how much money will it cost, if you have overlooked the early signs of tendon damage?). You must do this examination yourself.

Observe the horse's movement in order to see if and why it is lame.

The horse will try to avoid pain. If one leg hurts, the standing horse will take the weight off that leg, not place it flat on the floor or point it. If a horse points a foreleg, he is distributing his weight over the other three legs. If both forelegs hurt — such as with some forms of laminitis, the horse will point them forwards and bring his hind legs as far underneath him as he can, so that they take as much weight as possible. The movement of painful feet is restricted, so that weight is carried or the leg extended for as short a time as possible. Get an experienced person to lead the horse up in hand. He should hold the rope at about 40cm, walk next to the horse and look in the direction he wishes to go. (Always lead with a rope, of course, and not just by the headcollar; if the rope has a panic clasp, pull the rope through the headcollar once so that it doesn't open at the wrong moment; horses of which you are not certain should be lead in a bridle, with a bit or a chain.) If he holds the rope too short or if he walks in front of the horse, he will get in the way of both the horse's movement and your line of vision. When leading a horse, always look in the direction you wish the horse to travel — just as you would when riding. You often see people struggling to load a horse onto a trailer, because the person is standing on the ramp pulling on the rope and looking the horse directly in the eye. It would be absolutely illogical and unnatural if a horse allowed itself to be loaded in this way. Horses who load like this are sufficiently tolerant and far-sighted to overlook the weaknesses of their humans and to do what is required, even with the wrong instructions.

Watch the horse in walk and then in trot. Always look from the front, from the back and from the side. Lameness in the forelimbs can best be observed from the front. The horse will put more weight for longer on the sound leg. The horse will fall on the sound foot and nod (if he has enough length of rope) on the painful one. So if he falls on the offside, the lameness will be on the near side. Lameness behind is best observed from behind. The croup on the sound side will drop correspondingly lower. Watch, too, for whether the feet are pointed straight forward. Where the lameness is in the shoulder or the elbow, it can look as if the leg is being bent out and round (dishing). Lameness in the knee will often mean that the horse is reluctant to step backward. Check for a balanced diagonal across the back in trot. Lameness of the off hind leg will be compensated by the near fore. Seen from the front, this can look as if the horse is lame on the near fore (the horse falls on the front offside). Use your ears, too. The step on the sound leg is louder. Be aware of whether the lameness increases or reduces with movement.

As a further exercise, and if you have had a lot of practice, compare the lameness on hard and soft ground. Observe the difference in the lameness on left and right bends.

Horses whose cause of lameness is in the hoof or the joints generally go better on soft ground.

Lameness which originates far down in the leg (weight-bearing lameness) can be better seen on a circle, if the lame leg is on the inside. Lameness which originates higher up in the leg can be better seen on a circle with the lame leg on the outside. Of course, all this is quite complicated, and there are always exceptions. If in doubt, seek professional help.

Special examinations for suspected colic

Establish the pulse and respiratory rates, and take the temperature. Look at the mucous membranes and note the colour and dehydration. Check capillary filling time.

Look at the outside of the abdomen, particularly at whether it is unusually swollen or asymmetrical. With some forms of colic, the caecum becomes filled with gas, and the horse appears to be fatter on the right-hand side than on the left. If the pain is severe, the abdomen will be drawn up, the horse will appear to be thinner and the line of the muscle will be visible (tucked up). With a stallion, check whether the testicles are moving freely in the scrotum; in a mare, check for signs of pregnancy. Heavily pregnant mares sometimes present signs of low-grade colic when the foal is awake and practising piaffe or other movements. Without looking at the teats, labia and pelvic ligament, it is impossible to tell the difference between colic and the onset of labour.

Listen into your horse. This needs practice, too, so that you will know the quality and levels of normal digestive noise. If you lean your ear against the stomach, you will probably hear even better than with a stethoscope. Put your ear close to the left flank. There should be rumbling, liquid noises and perhaps also some higher sounds. At the lower left-hand part of the abdomen, the rumbling sounds should be similar. The sounds may also be a little deeper. At the lower right-hand part of the abdomen, first and foremost you should hear caecal noises, fermenting and rumbling. In the right flank there should be a splashing noise. At this point, your ear is near the point at which the small intestine meets the caecum. Around twice in a three-minute period, digested food should pass through this opening. The sounds associated with this process sounds similar to a toilet being flushed. If the sounds you hear are different, or if there is no splashing noise, it is not good. It is worse if you can hear nothing at all. A horse's digestive process is not regular. With colic, it is a question of collecting symptoms. If your horse is behaving normally, producing droppings and eating with relish, then the absence of one type of noise is not necessarily a sign of trouble.

3 Bandaging

Generally speaking, you will need help applying a bandage. Ideally, there will be two other people: one to hold the bandages and the other to pass them to you. When bandaging a hoof, the leg must be held up. All other bandages are better applied while the horse is standing on the affected leg. If there are several injuries, or fractures and fissures are involved, ensure that the horse is not required to bear weight. In such cases, you absolutely must not lift any of the other legs. In all other cases, however, the horse should be standing on the leg which is to be bandaged. If the horse doesn't agree, then a foreleg bandage should be applied whilst holding up the opposite leg. For a bandage to a hind leg, the foreleg on the same side should be held.

Bandaging the hoof/poulticing

A square cloth will always form the basis for a hoof bandage – a towel, cloth or a piece of cotton wool. Depending on what sort of bandage

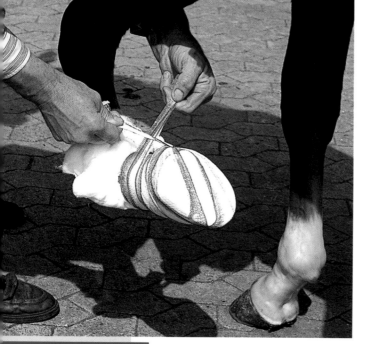

A bandage can be made out of a thick pad and baling twine.
Photo: Dr. Ende

you wish to apply, the cloth will be applied dry (for covering wounds or padding), or wet as a poultice (for packing bleeding hoof wall wounds or piercing injuries), or filled with bran (for treating bruising or so-called hoof abscesses) or ice packs (for cooling, in cases of laminitis, for example).

First, fold the cloth into a triangle. If you are going to use the cloth as a poultice, place the filling in the middle of the triangle. Get someone to lift the leg and hold it from the front. Apply the cloth with the long side at the back (and the corresponding right-angle at the front) to the underside of the hoof. Fold the corners over and/or around the hoof. Keep the poultice in place by wrapping a self-adhesive elastic bandage around the hoof. Try to bandage over and beyond the coronary band, which should be padded – generally speaking, the cloth will be large enough to accommodate this. Your helper who is holding the foot could help further by holding the end of the bandage in the pastern area (with his thumb). Then, when you have wrapped the bandage around the hoof a few times, you can bring it over the end and pull it straight over the tip of the hoof. Otherwise, bandaging the tip and the sole of the hoof is difficult. Once you have created a neat, colourful, hoof-shaped lump, you can set the foot down. Be careful, some horses are frightened by their odd-looking new foot or the sudden strange feeling. Be ready for the horse to lurch forward when the foot touches the ground. Be ready, too, for your bandage to fly off at the

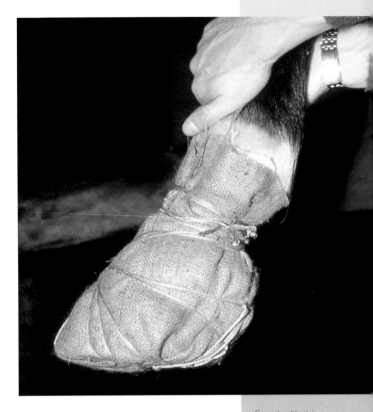

Correct support is obtained by the upper layer of sacking and additional twine. Photo: Dr. Ende

same time. Don't get cross. Rewind the bandage and start again. Check that the bandage is firmly in place without being too tight over the coronary band. You should be able to insert a finger between the coronary band and the bandage. If you are pleased with the bandage, you can reinforce the tip and the sole with sticky tape.

Bandaging the leg

Here, it is vitally important to use enough padding. However, knowing how much is enough is not so easy. If you pull the padding too tight, pressure points will be created, which can cause tissue damage. If it is too loose, it will fall off and lose its function,

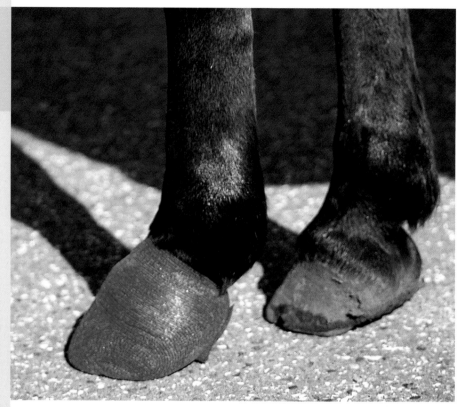

A triangular cloth under an elastic bandage is just as simple and holds equally well.
Photo: Würtz

and possibly also create further pressure points if it slips down.

If you need to cover a wound, you should apply a sterile non-adhesive dressing the correct way up (usually with the shiny side against the wound).

Try not to touch either the wound itself or the shiny side of the dressing, which will come into contact with the wound. If you drop the dressing, get a clean one.

Wrap two layers of gamgee or three layers of cotton wool around the leg. This type of bandage can be applied between the coronary band and just under the knee on a foreleg (under the hock for a hind leg).

The elastic self-adhesive bandage is needed to hold the whole thing in place. Roll out the bandage in such a way that the roll itself does not come between the unrolled part of the bandage and the leg, but lies on the outside. Unwind a small piece and lay it on the leg. That way, you will have more control over the pressure of the bandage than if you were to unroll the bandage directly around the leg. Start in the middle of the cannon bone, unroll and wrap the bandage gently and evenly downwards, overlapping the previous layer by about a third each time. Leave about 1cm of padding showing below the bottom of the bandage. If you are using cheap bandages or reusing a bandage which has already been used several times, the end will have to be taped.

It is, of course, possible to make bandages out of towels and gauze or stable bandages and plastic bags. However, without practice it is virtually impossible. An emergency situation is no time to be fighting with unsuitable materials, and this type of bandage simply does not hold up as well. If a horse tries to eat the bandages, the padding which has been left visible at the top and bottom should be bandaged in. A layer of creosote over the top will make the bandage unpalatable.

If you are intending to apply a pressure pad to a bleeding wound, then speed is of the essence. You will still need padding. You should apply an additional pressure pad over the padding (roll of cotton wool, packet of tissues or similar) at the appropriate point and apply the bandage tightly; if necessary, turn it over itself once. If blood seeps through the bandage, leave it in place and apply more pressure by applying another bandage over it. Use coloured bandages, simply because they look less dramatic than blood-soaked white ones.

Even with practice, bandages applied at the fetlock and hock are always difficult. First, apply a bandage over the cannon bone area on which the bandage on the joint can be supported. Apply plenty of padding over the bones. Stability will be most easily achieved if you wrap the bandage above and below the joint eight turns at a time – not too tight – and cross over from front to back and from back to front on the inside of the joint.

If you only want to bandage an

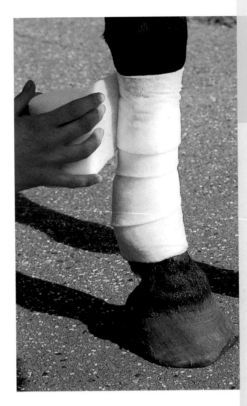

Bandage around the cannon bone. Good padding with cotton wool or similar is important.
Photo: Würtz

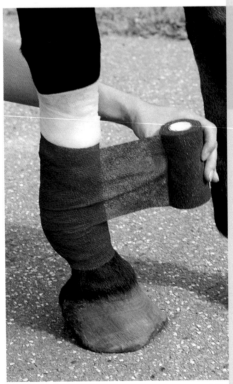

An elastic self-adhesive bandage is applied, not too tightly, around the outside.
Photo: Würtz

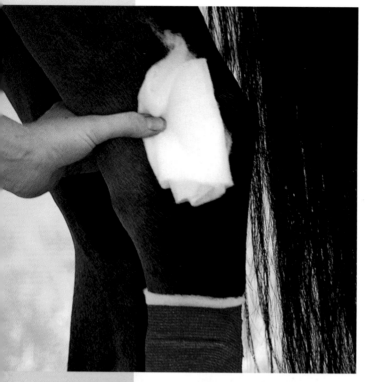

injured joint for a short period, disposable nappies soaked in antiseptic solution are suitable. They hold moisture and have their own self-adhesive fastenings.

Bandaging the head

Applying bandages which stay in place on the head is virtually impossible for the lay person, and a workable theoretical description is not easy, either. If you ever need such a bandage, to protect an eye, for example, get your vet to show you, or buy some special caps which are available on the market for just that purpose.

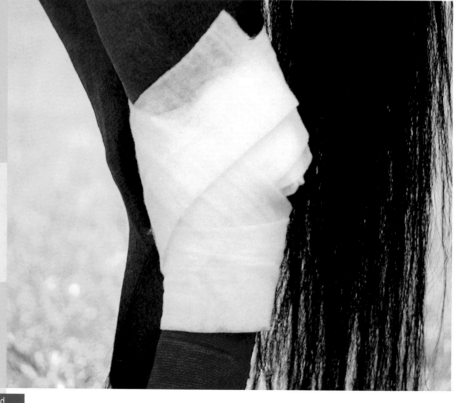

When bandaging the hock, a support bandage should first be applied to the cannon bone. Then ensure that the point of the hock and the Achilles' tendon lie between the padding in such a way that there is no pressure on them.
Photo: Würtz

This padding has already been fixed in place with the cotton wool. Each section of bandage is wrapped around eight times.
Photo: Würtz

4 Applying Forcible Measures

It is nicer if forcible measures do not have to be applied. Sadly, it is not always possible to do without. On the one hand, they may be necessary in order to treat a frightened or unwilling horse and, on the other hand, the dangers which a horse poses to both the helper and the vet can be considerable. If forcible measures are to be applied, then they must be applied knowledgeably and appropriately. In any case, a few minutes with a nose twitch is far better for the horse than hours of struggling.

In principle, just holding a horse is already a forcible measure of a kind, as is holding him by a bridle, a chain through the mouth or a chiffney bit. Another forcible measure is the holding up of one leg. What all these measures have in common is that they only hurt if the horse fights them.

Only use forcible measures on your vet's advice. If you need a twitch to take your horse's temperature every

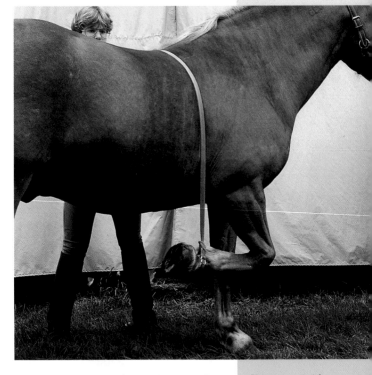

Using a rope to pick up a foreleg is easier, and kinder to the holder's back.
Photo: Dr. Ende

day or leave it on for an hour and a half while you are clipping him, perhaps you should think about taking the time to teach him to stand quietly, or only attempt such feats with the help of another person. Horses can get used to (almost) anything.

A very gentle method of applying such force is pressure massage on so-called sedation points. Find out where these are from an acupuncturist, or attend an acupuncture course. Rubbish? Not really. A lot of people use this type of manipulation intuitively and without realising it. Rubbing the forehead, for example, forms part of the way many riders praise/stroke their horses on a daily basis. Vets use it before and during dentistry treatment, Linda Tellington-Jones uses it in her teaching videos, as do Monty Roberts and others.

This is how to apply and hold a rope nose twitch.
Photo: Würtz

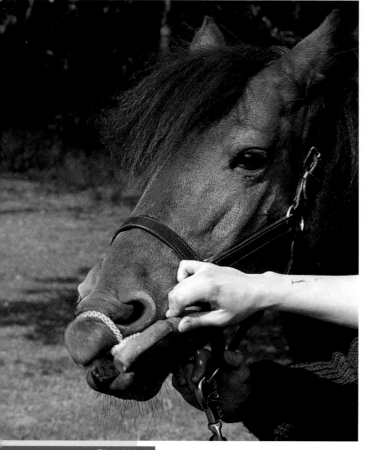

The nose or upper lip twitch

Rumour has it that nose twitches do not work, or not solely, by concentrating pain on the nose. The upper lip contains points which, when mechanically stimulated, release endorphins, or "happy messages". This is true. Knead your own upper lip between two fingers. After about twenty seconds you will feel more energetic. Some diets recommend this form of manipulation of the upper lip twenty minutes before eating, in order to reduce appetite. It is sensible, therefore, to apply the twitch and give it time to work before starting work on the horse again. This also means that the twitch should not be overly tight, because this only increases the pain (which provides a distraction from the other pain, which can also be useful, but generally speaking, light pressure will suffice). Gently moving a twitch which has not been jammed on will be more effective than pulling it tight.

The best form of twitch is the upper lip twitch made of wood and rope. The chains, wire, string and metal twitches used on cattle have no place on the upper lips of horses. The twitch should only be used on the upper lip and nowhere else!

When applying the twitch, hold it in your left hand (if you are right handed, hold it in your right hand) and reach through the loop. Let the loop hang across your hand between your third and little fingers.

This is because otherwise, when you go to grasp the lip, the twitch

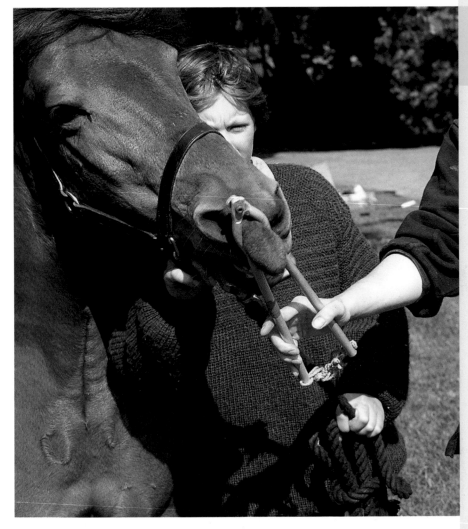

*Some horses respond
better to a metal twitch
like this one.
Photo: Würtz*

will slip over your wrist toward your elbow, and you will have to fish for it awkwardly. Thus armed, slowly, gently and talking calmly to your horse, reach from the left to the top of the nose. Let your hand lie there for a moment, then stroke gently down toward the top lip and grasp it gently. Wait a moment. Now take hold of the wooden handle with your right hand. Twist the rope round just so far that it doesn't fall off and then release the upper lip. I hope you are still talking to your horse. If a second person can hold the horse by the headcollar while the twitch is being applied, so much the better. Otherwise, use your right hand to hold both the headcollar and the rope and take it with you during the changeover.

The twitch should be held throughout the treatment. If you are alone, you can rest the wooden handle inside the noseband of the headcollar.

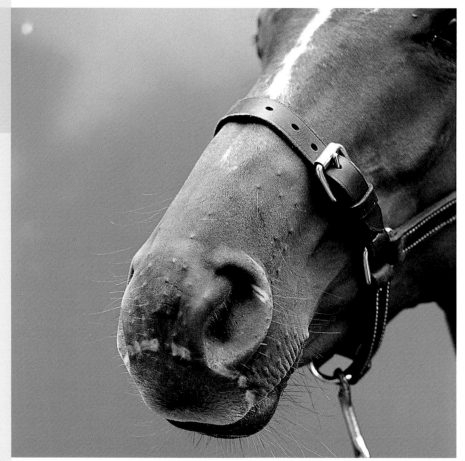

Restraining the horse

Some horses need to be restrained by tying up the back legs in order to prevent them bucking or kicking. This procedure is sometimes unavoidable when the vet is carrying out a rectal examination. It is also customary during covering.

To restrain the horse you will need a lunge rope, preferably a soft round rope, with no sharp edges. Make a loop and place it around the pastern area at the rear. If you are concerned about injury, you can wrap a small protective bandage around the foot. The lunge rope is then pulled along the horse's abdomen between the front legs and slung up around the neck to the other side. From the side of the leg to be tied up, grasp the lunge rope over the withers and make a quick release knot out of this end and the part of the rope that emerges through the front legs. Someone should hold the end of the lunge rope and be able to release it quickly in an emergency. After all, you don't want the horse to fall over. For the purpose of examination, it is generally sufficient to tie up a hind leg (the left leg, if the vet wishes to carry out the examination with his right hand).

5 How to Minimise the Risk of Injury

In any stable yard, the use of appropriate materials and safety should be a priority.

The bars of loose boxes should not be so far apart as to allow a foot to pass through. The walls should be sound and not bend or break if kicked. Stable doors should have secure locks and be kept closed. Where there are footbolts, these should also be kept closed. Feet jammed between the door and the sill when the top bolt is closed are a nightmare. However careful you are, accidents with insecurely closed stable doors happen time and again. Get organised, so that the last person to leave the yard at night checks that all the doors are securely closed. When a horse enters or leaves his stable, he should be wearing a headcollar and lead rope. You should walk into the stable in front of your horse. The unexpected can sometimes happen, even with the most well-accustomed and well-mannered of horses. It is

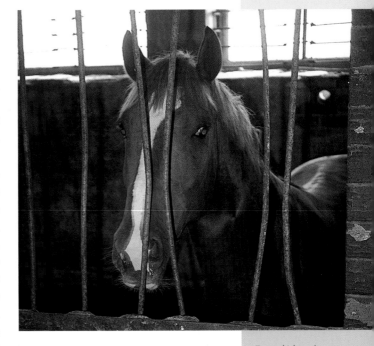

not possible to restrain a horse by the headcollar alone, and there is no chance at all if he has no headcollar on. In some yards, it is normal practice for a horse which has been standing tied up in the corridor to be tak-

Bars which are bent and widely spaced are enormously dangerous. It would be easy for a leg to pass between these bars, resulting in a serious injury. Photo: Dr. Ende

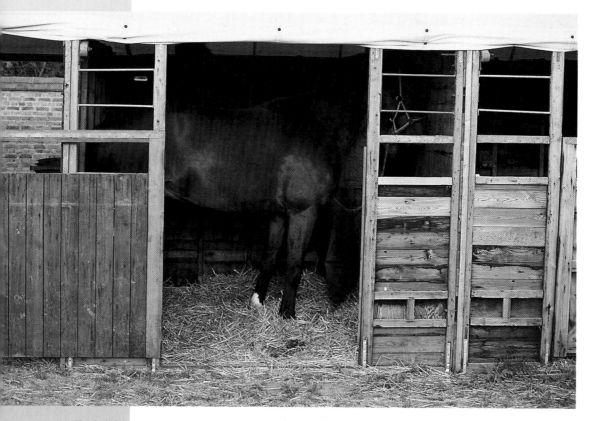

A stable which is clearly too small, such as this one, goes against the principles of animal welfare and poses a serious risk of casting.
Photo: Dr. Ende

en to the stable door on just a head-collar and released.

If he goes into the stable, he is rewarded with a cheerful slap on the rump. But what happens if he decides to go somewhere else? Or takes fright (because there's a monster in the stable)? With any luck, at least the barn or yard doors will be closed.

The floor outside the stable must always be safe to walk on. If you wash the horse's legs and then grease the hooves, things can get pretty slippery. There should be a designated washing area, and the area outside the stables should remain dry (you can sprinkle it with water to bind the dust before sweeping up, but should not wet it). Think before tipping out

even small amounts of water, especially in winter. It really is not necessary to tip a bucket of water across the yard on a winter's afternoon when the temperature is falling, because by the following morning you will have created a skating rink.

Headcollars should be well-fitting and, if horses are to wear them while unsupervised, made of breakable material. A good, solid nylon headcollar is of no use if the horse is likely to break before the headcollar does. A well-fitting headcollar sits close enough to the head so that the horse's own hind feet (scratching an ear), someone else's feet (playing) or someone else's teeth can't get hooked up in it, but it should also be loose enough not to leave marks on the hair. Leather headcollars are best. It is even better not to leave a horse unsupervised with a headcollar on.

For technical reasons, this is not possible in some yards, if the yard owner insists that horses may only be turned out with a headcollar, or if blinkers or fly-nets need to be attached. If headcollars are removed once the horses are in the field, they must be left somewhere where they can be easily found, but far enough away from the fence to avoid the horses pulling them into the field.

Only tie up your horse where there is a secure tying ring. Horses that run off still attached to the hitching rail, an old gate or the bike rack will injure themselves seriously.

Use quick-release knots, but tie them firmly. Panic clasps are not always the answer. If you lead a nervous horse on a panic clasp, it may be that one jump will be all it takes for the horse to get away. Teach your horse to stand quietly next to you without fidgeting, and to wait until you allow him to go through the gate and turn him toward you before letting him go into the field. Any other behaviour is irritating and is also dangerous for you both.

Use only the best quality headcollars, ropes, bridles, tack and girths, check them over regularly and take good care of them. Stirrup leathers which break, bandages which come undone and bridles and bits which break while in use pose a considerable risk.

When your horse is grazing in the field, it must be fenced in. The best fencing is, of course, wooden post and rail with electric tape along the

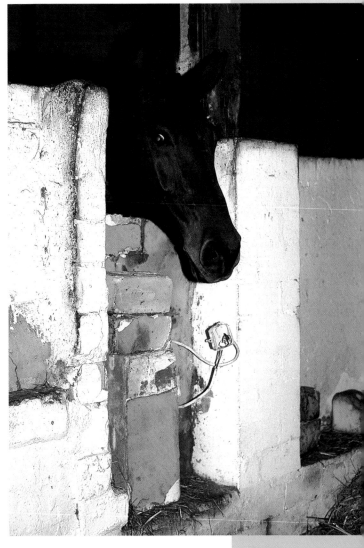

Accommodation like this is entirely unsuitable for horses, and is a considerable safety risk.
Photo: Dr. Ende

top or the side. Barbed wire has acquired a bad reputation because it can cause injuries which do not heal well. However, a tautly strung, properly maintained barbed wire fence is not the worst kind of fencing. More dangerous, but still in frequent use are plain wire (some of it electrified), electric tape which will not break in an emergency, rotten wood, sagging tape, broken plastic posts, metal rods and sheep wire. If electric tape or

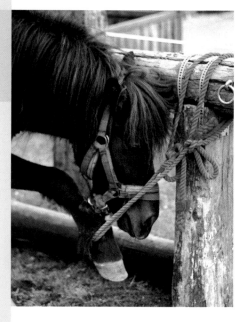

Never tie horses on too long a rope, or leave them tied up unsupervised.
Photo: Dr. Ende

Barbed wire should not be used as fencing for paddocks, as the risk of injury to horses is very high.
Photo: Dr. Ende

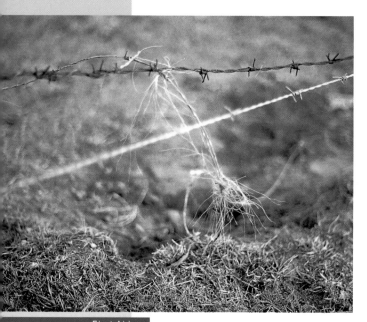

wire is used, it must be strung taut and be easy to maintain.

If a horse becomes tangled in fencing, the fencing should break before the horse's bones do. Electric fences should have a circuit breaker, so that they switch off automatically if a horse becomes tangled up, or they should be easy to switch off. The health of a horse which is caught in plain wire and receiving an electric shock every two seconds will be seriously at risk and it will be hard to free for as long as the electricity remains on. Wire cutters kept in the vicinity of all forms of wire fencing can be a life-saver.

Where possible, fences should be clearly visible and incorporate a visible obstacle: a kink, or a wall or hedge behind the fence make clearly visible obstacles. Fences should not be set directly adjacent to a ditch. Leave at least 3 metres between the fence and the ditch. It is hard enough to extract a horse from a ditch – but I deal with this elsewhere in this book.

Equestrian establishments should be fenced off from the road. Rather inconveniently, this will mean the installation of a gate, which not only has to be opened, but also closed and/or locked every time you ride through it. Doors to indoor and outdoor manèges and jumping arenas should also be kept closed.

No horse should ever be left on its own in a field, although there are a very few exceptions. The last horse must be brought in, even if this is not always simple. It is always better, of course, to go twice than to try to lead three horses. If you want to lead two horses together, always take the horse which is caught first up to the other one. Never, even for a moment, tie the first horse up to the fence or the gate. He may panic and take the fence or the gate with him. Do not open the gate until all the horses are under control. If you have a large group of horses, or if there are ponies

– past masters at slipping out unnoticed – make a corral inside the gate. Then, if another horse does get past you, at least it will still be contained.

All areas which are used by unsupervised horses should be free of rolls of wire, old rug straps, lunge ropes left lying around, bucket handles, jutting-out nails, hardcore, baling twine, wheel-barrows and other detritus.

Manèges should be regularly checked for and cleared of stones. All those useful items which you need for your horse should be kept out of his reach. Ropes and/or chains left hanging for tying up purposes should be so far out of reach as not to create a risk of strangling, should the horse pull it into the stable with him.

Horses should never be allowed to race off if their muscles and joints are cold. When we ride, we carefully warm them up for twenty minutes, so lead horses to the field yourself, or let them walk around for at least five minutes before letting them go. You risk injury if, in winter, you simply open the stable door and let all the horses rush out. The danger is even greater in the dim light of the early morning, when you can hardly see unlevel or stony ground. If the horses then jostle and trot about on a concrete yard before dashing off round a corner, you are asking for trouble. Driving lanes should be as well fenced as paddocks. Gates should be opened in the same way as lock gates. The drives out and home should never be totally uncontrolled. You cannot possibly hold up even well-mannered horses by yourself on a five-metre wide track if the whole herd

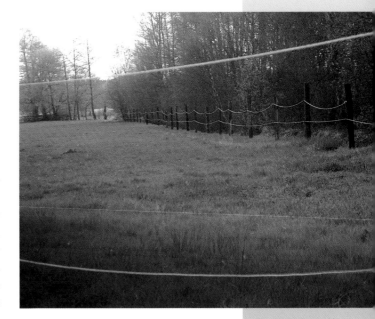

unexpectedly gallops back towards you because there are still ghosts lurking in the field.

It is sensible to turn out groups of horses together who know and like each other.

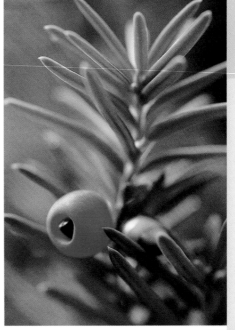

Fences must be suitable and regularly maintained. Sagging tapes like these are dangerous.
Photo: Dr. Ende

Yew is pretty, but very poisonous. Beare of its presence near paddocks.
Photo: Dr. Ende

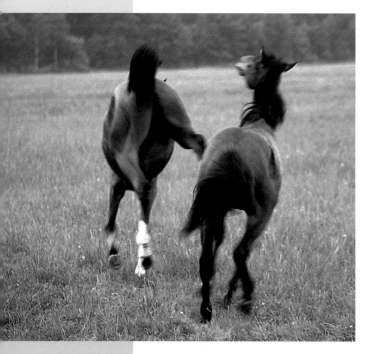

Even under the best conditions in a sufficiently large field, there is always a risk of injury, particularly with young horses. This is why, even at grass, horses must be checked every day.
Photo: Dr. Ende

For the sake of peace and harmony in the field, it may be that mares and geldings have to be separated. Each group should be kept as constant as possible in order to avoid fights over the pecking order. After riding or walking out together with a senior group member, new horses should be introduced by daylight and with some supervision. Perhaps the new horse could spend the first couple of nights in the stable next door to the head of the herd. It makes no sense to leave them together for a short period each evening, and immediately separate them every time they chase each other. It will cost you no end of nerves, and it only confuses the horses' natural getting-to-know-you games and prevents them from sorting out the pecking order. Give the new group time to get used to each other; they will not normally cause each other serious harm. Horses

which are new to a group, and those who like to kick, should have their back shoes removed.

When you are riding, be careful of your own safety by wearing suitable riding clothes and a protective riding hat, and by using good quality tack. Don't ride out alone, or, if you must, tell someone where you intend to go so that if you do have an accident, you can be found quickly. If your horse needs help, you will not be able to leave it. Take a mobile phone with you. You can always switch it off. In general, it is not necessary for a horse to wear protective boots when being ridden. If your horse forges or over-reaches, you will need overreach boots, or tendon boots if you intend to jump. Bandaging is less useful. Check your horse's general health and legs before you ride out. Pick out feet before and after riding.

If you ride out in a group, try to put horses together who like each other and riders who ride to a similar standard (riders are allowed to like each other, too, and I did not mean to say that you should always ride out with novices and leave the more advanced riders at home). Keep a sufficient distance between you at all paces, both at the side and to the rear. Only ride side-by-side if the paths allow, and pass any riders who come toward you left shoulder to left shoulder (you may greet them, too). When you are out riding, don't allow your horse to rub noses with, squeal or lash out with a foreleg at other horses, and always keep hold of your reins.

Of course, you can trundle along on a loose rein, but you must be able to return to the saddle and the position you were in if your horse spooks or shies. Practise new moves in the company of a more experienced horse and when you have plenty of time.

Make sure that you comply with the regulations governing bridleways and the Highway Code as it applies to horses.

If you are riding a path for the first time, stay in walk. If you have to cross water, be clear in your mind that you do not know what may be lying at the bottom. At the end of the winter, be particularly careful during a thaw; it may be that the bottom of deeper puddles is still frozen. Rather than experiment, dismount and lead your horse for a while, otherwise, you may be leading your poor, lame horse for weeks. This is particularly annoying if it is your own fault.

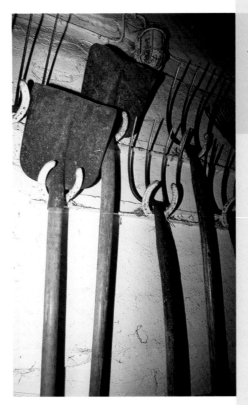

Perfect accommodation for yard tools. It is easily accessible, but at the same time will not get under anyone's feet. Foto: Dr. Ende

---

*CHECKLIST –
WHAT TO DO IN AN
EMERGENCY*

BEFORE
- *Improve immediate surroundings*
  - → *improveng fencing*
  - → *repair locks/bolts*
  - → *remove any nails which are sticking out*
  - → *build and use a gate to the road*
  - → *check tack*
  - → *check shoeing*
  - → *check condition of trailer*
  - → *check carefully whether all potential risks have been avoided*

- *Make a yard first aid kit*
- *Create a designated space*
  - → *designate treatment and farriery areas*
  - → *do not store forks, bicycles, rolls of wire or other rubbish in these areas*

- *Check headcollars and ropes*
  - → *well-fitting leather headcollars, thick ropes without quick-release clasps*

- *Wear practical clothing*
  - → *sensible footwear with non-slip soles – always*

- *Practise*
  - → *everything you might possibly need in an emergency*

→ *bandaging, taking temperature,
using a nose twitch and much else*

- *Train horses*
  → *This is a comprehensive task,
  which cannot be defined in terms of
  time.*
  → *If a horse will not pick up his feet,
  or will only do so under threat of
  violence, even a simple hoof abscess
  will not be easy to treat. If you are
  going to need two or three hours
  and at least five helpers in the
  middle of the night to load a horse
  with colic onto a trailer, then just
  the lost time could cost the horse his
  life. If your horse tries to bite vets,
  strangers or just men on principle,
  what might be regarded as an
  endearing little foible on a normal
  day could be quite a hindrance to
  treating him in an emergency.*

IN AN EMERGENCY

- *Keep calm*
- *Assess the situation*
- *Assess the patient*
- *Call or phone for help or get
  someone else to do it*
- *Delegate tasks, inform the
  owner of the horse (or get some-
  one else to do it)*
- *Give first aid*
- *Ensure that the process of res-
  cue and veterinary attention
  runs flawlessly*

AFTERWARDS

- *Take a deep breath*
- *Thank helpers, and make a
  note of addresses, if necessary*
- *Make a note of any damage*
- *Ask about the next steps with
  regard to treatment, feeding
  and movement of the horse*
- *Make an appointment for a
  follow-up visit*
- *Spend some time with the
  horse – tell him a story …*
- *Replenish the yard first aid kit*

6 Injuries

Establish the site and the extent of the injury on the horse. Where the site of an injury is extremely sensitive, such as the hoof wall and the pastern area, all joint areas and the head, even minor injuries should be thoroughly investigated. Small wounds at other sites which have not fully pierced the skin can be washed with clean water and covered with wound cream.

Important: make sure your horse's tetanus injections are up-to-date.

Injuries to the skin

Where there are gaping wounds and heavy bleeding, such as puncture wounds and wounds that have formed a pouch, veterinary help should always be sought. All wounds must be cleaned if they are to heal properly. Washing with clear or tepid salt water (one teaspoonful of salt to one litre of water) is indicated. Washing means no more than letting water pour over the wound. Use a hose to do this – sponges are not suitable. Touching the wound, poking about in it or similar actions will

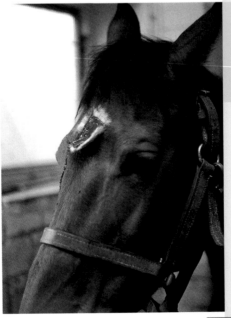

Head wounds are always dangerous and require veterinary attention.
Photo: Dr. Ende

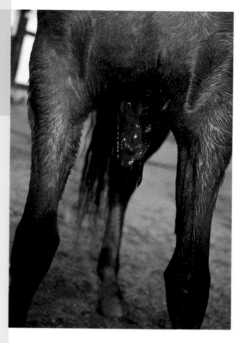

Injuries like this should be presented to the vet as fresh as possible, so that they can be stitched. Photo: Dr. Ende

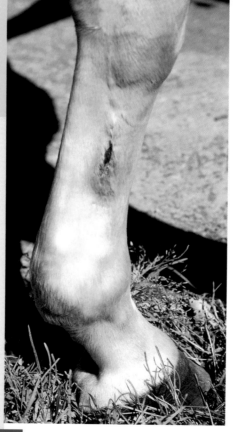

Even a little scratch like this is no mere bagatelle. If it is not attended to, it will cause problems at the latest within 24 hours. Photo: Dr. Ende

only increase the risk of allowing dirt or bacteria to enter it.

Care needs to be taken where the wound has formed a pouch: ensure that dirt and dried blood is washed out, not in. Rinsing the affected area with water will also give a clearer view. Any wounds which are to receive veterinary attention should not have anything put into them. Once you have washed the wound, dress it with clean, soft cloths or bandage it. Your only aim is to avoid further damage and dirt until the vet arrives. If you apply wound powder or disinfectant spray, you could be delaying the healing process, obscuring the vet's view of the wound or even making stitching impossible.

Take a good look at the wound. What looks like a small scratch could be a puncture wound, or even contain a foreign body (a splinter or similar). If all you do is put wound cream on it, you may get a nasty surprise the following morning when the whole leg is swollen and the horse is unable to put any weight on it. At this point, you must call the vet. If in doubt, ask. A competent riding instructor and/or yard owner will be able to advise you whether to call the vet. It is always better to call the vet once too often.

Joint injuries

Injuries in joint areas require special care. If a joint has been injured, there will usually be a flow of synovial fluid. The wound secretion will be yellowish in colour and may be frothy.

If you take some between your fingers, it should be stringy. If this is what you find, tell your vet when you call him. Be particularly careful in covering such wounds – it is best to use the sterile dressings from the yard first aid kit. Do not move the horse – at all.

Closed joint injuries are sprains or twists. The joint will swell and the horse will be unable to move it, or only with difficulty. He will be obviously lame. You can hose it with cold water, or apply an ice pack until the vet arrives.

If a joint makes a creaking sound, this can be an indication of bleeding.

Heavy bleeding

The first thing to be done is to stop the bleeding as rapidly as possible. Tying off the injured area towards the heart is often described, but is rarely successful. If you tie off too tightly or for too long, you can cause considerable damage. Arterial bleeding, when the blood spurts out from the wound in pulses, is the only time when tying off can be justified. In that event, try to find a well-muscled area further up the leg and apply the tourniquet at that point. Cushion the tourniquet with at least a towel in order to avoid it causing further injury. Never leave a tourniquet on for more than twenty minutes and, if necessary, loosen it for a minute and then reapply.

In almost every case of heavy bleeding, it is better to apply firm pressure yourself.

A pressure bandage should be applied to lower leg areas. Apply a

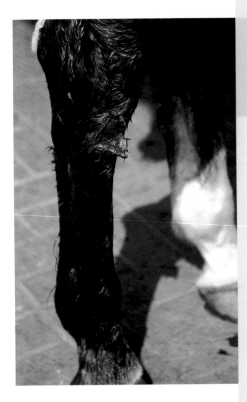

Deep wounds which are also near a joint require veterinary attention.
Photo: Dr. Ende

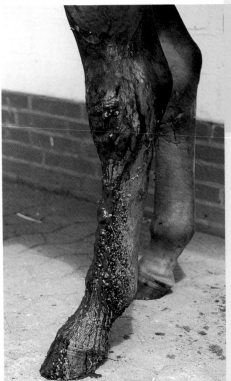

Once the vet has been called, the wound can be washed with clear water, so that you can see how bad the wound really is.
Photo: Dr. Ende

non-adhesive dressing to the wound and quickly wrap gamgee and an elastic bandage around it. You can incorporate a second dressing into the elastic bandage over the wound area (gamgee, a packet of paper tissues or something similar). This first bandage may well become blood-soaked. Don't panic. Do not remove this bandage, but apply another bandage over the top, again with padding over the wound for reinforcement.

On all other areas of the body, you will have to try to stem the bleeding by pressing clean cloths, cotton wool or similar items firmly over the bleeding vessel. The horse's blood pressure will decrease with the blood loss, and your chance of stemming the flow will increase accordingly.

Try to objectively assess the amount of blood lost. A large horse can lose up to ten litres before the situation becomes really precarious. A litre of blood, which doesn't look much contained in a bucket, looks like an incredible amount when spilt all over the yard.

Flesh wounds

In most cases, flesh wounds bleed moderately, look awful and should always be stitched. Transport to the nearest veterinary clinic and an anaesthetic are frequently unavoidable. Above all, ensure that the horse is prevented from taking care of his wound himself. If a wound is irritating them, horses tend to try to bite or rub it. Both will introduce dirt into the wound. Get someone to hold the horse or tie him up short. Do not wash out the wound. It can be difficult to see the extent of such wounds, and there may be a considerable risk of penetrating deeper into it. The bleeding will clean the wound, you should merely cover it to keep it clean. If there is a lot of blood, apply pressure by pressing dressings, cotton wool or towels into the wound.

Wounds containing foreign bodies

If you see something sticking out of a wound, it is a very natural reaction to want to pull it out. Stop, however, and think.

Injuries on the torso which have pieces of wood jutting out of them may become even more dramatic as soon as the wood is removed, since a possible consequence would be heavy bleeding and a prolapse of the organs of the abdominal cavity. Keep the horse calm and wait for the vet.

With injuries to the rib-cage, the foreign body will automatically seal the puncture point. If you remove it, however well-meaning your action, air will get into the puncture, the lung will collapse and you will not be able to close the hole as fast as either you would wish or is necessary.

Generally, you will have discovered the injured horse, so you will not know the size of the foreign body, or how deep it has penetrated.

If the situation is uncertain, it may be better to wait until the vet, an anaesthetic and stitching equipment have arrived before removing the foreign body.

Foreign bodies can be removed from the legs immediately. Make a note of the site and depth of the wound. Keep the foreign body, and consider whether anything could be left in the wound. This could easily be the case with rotten wood, for example.

You may think that this is all a bit exaggerated, but I have encountered some really unimaginable cases a wooden fence post in an abdomen (ultimately fatal); a splinter of hoof in a hind leg following a kick (unfortunately also fatal); a pine needle in the coronary band (found while trimming the foot after weeks of going unlevel); glass splinters in the chest muscle following an accident with a car (these worked themselves out four years after the accident and the horse experienced no problems in the intervening time); a section of a wire bucket handle in a hoof (the wire was surgically removed and healed without complications); small pieces of wire from a barbed wire fence following an injury (discovered in the hock by an X-ray taken some months later; the horse presented no symptoms).

Injuries to the hoof wall and foreign bodies in the hoof

It is possible for the hoof wall to shatter merely by the horse knocking it against a stone lying in its path while walking. Both the pain and the risk of residual damage to the horse are considerable. Generally speaking, the horse cannot put any weight on the foot, and there is heat. The pulsa-

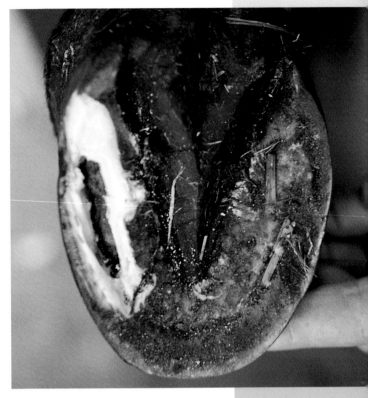

Here a ripe abscess within the hoof wall has been lanced. This is commonly referred to as a hoof abscess. Photo: Dr. Ende

tion of the digital artery is clear. Put a bandage on and call the vet and the farrier.

With injuries to the sole, you will initially need only the bandage and the vet. If there are still objects in the hoof and you are unable to assess the size of them, consider the following:

The soft parts of the hoof, into which nails and similar objects can easily penetrate, lie directly above sensitive structures, which are difficult to see. If you can see a piece of a metal object, such as the head of a nail, in the area of the corner of the heel or frog cleft, it may be that the rest of the object has insulted the navicular bursa.

An X-ray taken before removing the object would certainly confirm this. However, if you are miles from

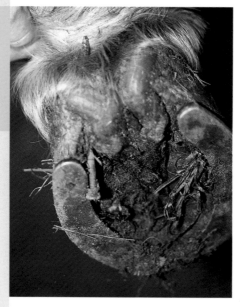

It is rare for a puncture wound to be as obvious as this. Often, only a very small piece of the foreign body is visible.
Photo: Dr. Ende

the nearest electrical socket, you will have to remove the object yourself. This may not be as simple as it sounds. If necessary, use a pair of pliers (which, of course, you will always have to hand – from now on you will only ride out fully equipped with a first-aid kit and toolbox). Bandage the foot and call the vet. As I said earlier, it is better to call the vet once

too often, as the following example shows:

A horse treads on a nail. It is clearly visible and is obviously causing problems, so it is removed by a well-meaning person. To the horse's – and the person's – relief everything seems to be fine and the horse is allowed to stay in the field. Everything still looks fine the next day. Three days later, the horse is unwilling to put any weight on the foot, in fact it is reluctant to put any weight on either foreleg. Now, which foot was the puncture in – right or left? In any event, the horse is taken to the nearest veterinary clinic, where the wound is immediately treated under anaesthetic, but sadly days too late. There are maggots in the navicular bursa and the other hoof is showing signs of laminitis as a consequence of excessive weight-bearing. There is nothing to be done.

Injuries to tendons and ligaments

Lameness which sets in suddenly because of injured tendons and ligaments is usually the result of damage caused by overloading, the signs of which have been coming on slowly and unnoticed for a few days. Take the time to check the condition of your horse's legs every day. Don't ignore small changes, swellings or heat in the legs.

If you suddenly have an obvious problem, lameness and so-called "bowed" tendons, do not move your horse more than is absolutely necessary.

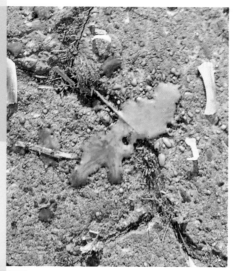

The pressure built up by the pus running out with blood and decomposing horn was so intense that, prior to lancing, the horse was severely lame.
Photo: Dr. Ende

In any event, this type of change is most frequently noticed just before a ride. Call the vet. In the initial stages, damage to the tendon sheath can be confused with damage to the actual tendon, although it is much less harmful. Your vet will be able to assess the site, size and extent of the damage by palpation or an ultrasound scan. The result of this will affect the treatment, healing time and the scope for work afterwards. Some tendon injuries never heal, so that the horse can return to full work, and because the structures are under considerable pressure and subject to poor circulation, healing tends to be very slow. Modern veterinary medicine has a number of better and faster healing methods at its disposal than before, but the fundamental principle remains: tendons need rest to heal. Feed supplements, injections, bandaging and orthopaedic measures support the healing process but unless sufficient time is allowed, they can do nothing. Depending on the damage done, sufficient time can mean anything between four weeks and twelve months. Under no circumstances should you try to start work again too early. Relapses are worse and take longer.

If the damage occurs far from home or, typically, on a Sunday and you cannot or do not wish to call the vet immediately, you can do the right thing by putting the horse on box or paddock rest and by using a bandage with aremorica powder or an ice-pack.

Tendon damage can also, of course, be the result of trauma. The classic

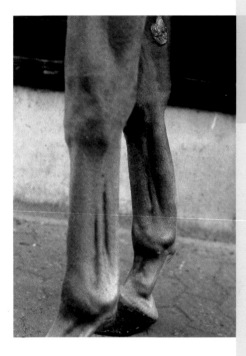

This picture shows a so-called bowed tendon, a swelling in the area of the flexor tendons
Photo: Dr. Ende

scenario is the broken-down race-horse which can be acquired cheaply and which has every chance of giving many years of service, but he must be given time.

Equally common are injuries caused by a foot going down a rabbit hole or similar. In these cases, there is significant bleeding at the points where the sinews are torn and the area swells visibly. Keep the horse still until the vet arrives, in any event, it will be unlikely to want to walk. A tearing tendon makes a cracking noise, which can be clearly heard if you are in the vicinity.

The prognosis for open tendon injuries, such as a flexor tendon in the foreleg after being struck by a swinging, steel-clad hind foot, is not at all favourable. Cover the wound, keep the patient calm, stay where you are and wait for the vet.

Avulsion injuries, known as insertion desmopathy (at the suspensory ligament or the accessory ligament of the deep digital flexor tendon) can be caused by short-term strain. They can be diagnosed precisely by ultrasound scan, and heal very slowly.

Muscle injuries

Pulled muscles and muscle fibres are caused by impact injuries, road traffic accidents and strain. Significant swelling of the muscle belly occurs rapidly. Pain can appear to be considerable (upper and lower arm, lower thigh) or slight (abdominal wall). The swelling is warm and initially feels as if it is filled with liquid; later it becomes tight and solid. It is painful to the touch. Cold compresses on the affected area can bring relief. Later on, when the initial bleeding has been stemmed, creams containing heparin will help. You can get these from your vet.

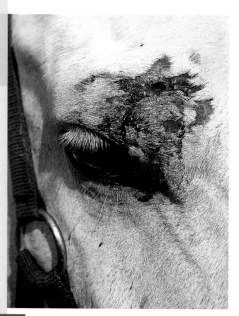

Injury directly adjacent to the eye. Photo: Dr. Ende

As with swelling and bruising, the application of a packet of frozen peas will help. This is a cheap, non-toxic remedy that has no doping effects. Larger bleeds can be aspirated later if resorption is insufficient. Aspiration will only be effective from ten days after the accident.

Eye injuries

Generally, it is only the area around the eye which is injured. Veterinary attention is always required, because otherwise diffuse abscesses can occur. Since the injury will irritate the horse, it will rub the area around its eye and cause considerable additional damage. You should prevent this.

Injuries to the edge of the eyelid absolutely must be treated surgically. Otherwise the eyelid will not shut properly and the result will be a lifetime of problems. Generally, this type of surgery will be carried out at the veterinary clinic. However, if you are lucky, it can be done at home under local anaesthetic without sedation.

If the eye itself is injured, it will water and the surface of the cornea will have a bumpy appearance. It may become clouded. It will turn grey if the moisture content increases. The cornea will spring up around the defect. Your vet will establish whether the cornea itself has been injured or even become separated This will require examination with a special light, which will also be able to determine whether the pupil is open or closed.

It is not good for the pupil to

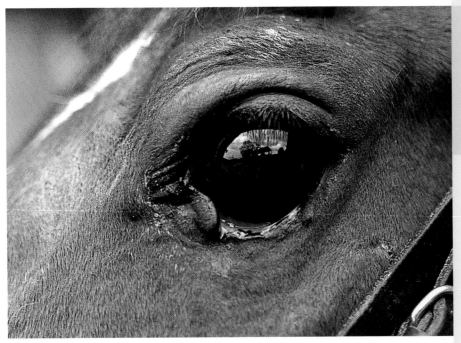

remain closed for any length of time, because adhesions can form in this part of the eye. It may be that fluorescin drops – a dye which marks the defect – will need to be used in order to establish the full extent of the injury. Following an application of atropine ointment, the pupil should open after about twenty minutes, and the effect should last for several days. This means, above all, that the dosage does not need to be repeated. The atropine will also relieve the pain to some degree.

Eye injuries are very painful and your horse will need medication.

Acute conjunctivitis looks dramatic. The eyes will stream with tears as a result of periodic infection and here, too, urgent veterinary attention is required.

Ask someone to show you how to apply eye ointment to the eye. The tube should not come into contact with the eye – after all, you are trying to treat an injury, not create a new one. Eye medications are sterile, so applying them with your fingers is no good. Open tubes should not be left lying around. Never use old tubes of ointment.

Ointment will often have to be

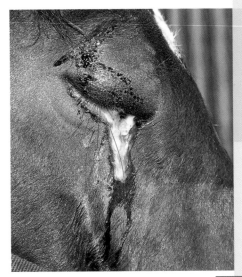

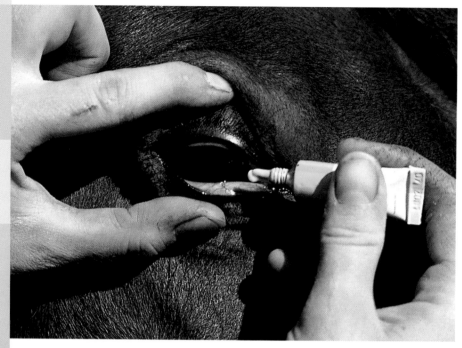

Carefully drop oint-
ment into the lower
conjunctival sac. The
tube should not touch
the eye. For safety,
always get someone else
to hold the horse.
Photo: Würtz

The ointment will
then distribute itself
over the whole surface
of the eye. This will
give your horse an eery
look, but that's how it
should be.
Photo: Würtz

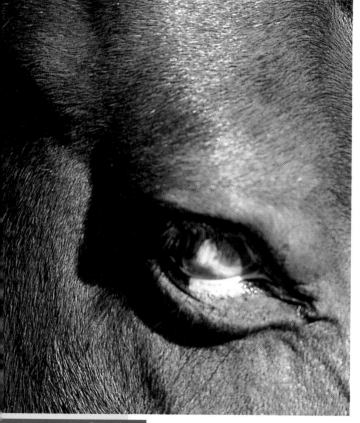

applied several times a day, sometimes even hourly. Show everyone
involved exactly what to do, when
and where.

You can remove foreign bodies
from the eye yourself. When riding
through rough countryside, tiny
thorns may get into the horse's eye.
Removal is recommended in every
case. The small channel formed by
the removal will usually close by
itself. However, you should, of
course, call the vet once the object
has been removed.

Injured or sore eyes can be lightly
covered with a damp cloth until the
vet arrives. Applying a head bandage
is not easy and generally not a task
for the layman. You can put on
ready-made eye covers, which are
available commercially.

Horses with eye problems should
not be exposed to direct sunlight
outside, or to draughts or dust inside.

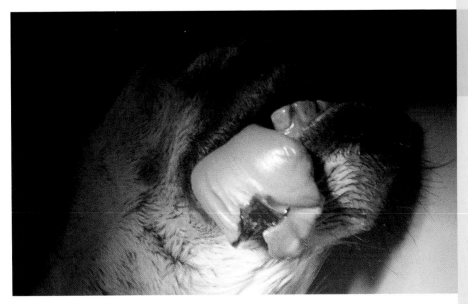

Tongue injuries

When horses play together, it sometimes happens that they injure their tongues. Similar injuries can be caused by enemies attacking each other through the bars of loose boxes. Tongues need to be intact. Take the horse to the veterinary clinic and let it be treated with surgery. It is wrong to assume that "It'll be OK". Foreign bodies in the mouth cavity and the tongue will prevent the horse from eating properly. If he does not want to take a treat and is not otherwise showing signs of colic, have a look in his mouth (even if he was a gift!). Splinters of wood can become lodged at the base of the tongue, far back in the mouth and near to the teeth. You will only be able to see them if you open the mouth with a Houseman's gag and use a torch. Excessive salivation can also be a sign of injuries in the mouth cavity. Infected tongues can swell and protrude between the front teeth.

By way of example, a horse which bites a piece out of his cheek in a fall should also be taken to the veterinary clinic.

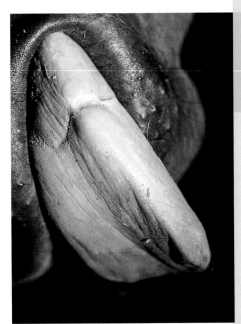

7 Nosebleeds

A nosebleed can occur once in a lifetime, or it can happen time and time again. Following an injury to the ethmoid bone, bleeding can be severe. If the horse is over-exerted, the lungs may bleed, causing bright red blood to flow out of the nose.

In the space of fifteen minutes, a horse can easily lose a quarter of a litre of blood through his nose. Place a bucket under his nose, so that you can assess the quantity. Hold the head low. After two or three litres, you should call the vet if the bleeding has not reduced. If your horse has several nosebleeds, he should be thoroughly examined.

Here, a little pale coloured blood is running from both nostrils. Presumably, this is a reaction to the horse's earlier exertions.
Photo: Dr. Ende

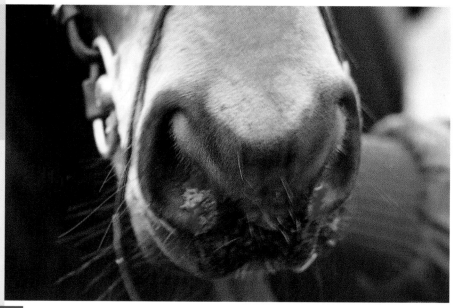

8 Splints

Splints are always a sudden discovery. Understandably, it is usually assumed that "he must have been kicked", which is quite possible. However, young horses often present with splints on the inside of the cannon bone during their early training. If too much is demanded of them, these horses, whose balance under the rider has not yet been perfected, stand with their legs apart and cause compression injuries to the structures joining the cannon and splint bones. When it is overtaxed, the horse's body feels the need to calcify and develop more bone at this point. The splint we see is damage caused by over-exertion. Only work your horse in accordance with its strength and level of training.

If a splint has formed as a result of over-exertion, and your horse is not lame, you can treat it yourself. Rest is most important in order to prevent further (over-)reaction. Soak a sponge in a mixture of cider vinegar and water (1:1). Place the sponge on the splint and bandage with a stable bandage and padding. Leave at least overnight, and for about the next five nights.

Splints can also form as a result of kicks and injuries to the thin skin over the bone. The body will then form more bone. Fresh splints require rest, otherwise they will grow and grow and end up looking like cauliflowers. Old, flat splints are mostly just unsightly. Pay attention to whether a splint is likely to cause pressure on any important structures either now or in the future.

Open splints

Following an injury, changes sometimes occur which feel like splints and on which there is a small open wound.

Treatment should be sought immediately. X-rays may be necessary immediately and later on. Despite treatment, the lump is often permanent and the wound heals well initially, but never quite completely. Your horse should have been X-rayed by this time. This type of injury causes sequestrum, and chips of bone which form under the skin but are not joined to the actual bone. These will cause lifelong problems and must be surgically removed. Generally, this will mean a stay at the veterinary clinic and full anaesthesia.

9 Fractures

It is no longer the case that a broken leg signs a horse's death warrant. Modern surgical techniques, physiotherapy and medicines mean that there are far greater possibilities now than even a few years ago.

Not every fracture which heals successfully will guarantee a return to soundness and full performance, which is why a mare with good papers is likely to have more chance of living on than a gelding. Fractures are costly and time-consuming and, sadly, nowadays few are prepared to do this for a horse which will be useless. Then there is the animal welfare aspect – how much pain and impairment can you reasonably expect a horse to bear?

Horses with fractures to weight-bearing limb bones will generally not put the affected leg down. Do not, under any circumstances, give painkillers or attempt to move the horse.

A small fissure can easily turn into

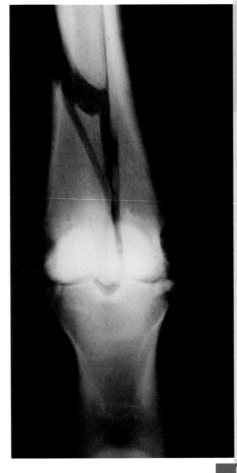

An X-ray will show the nature and extent of a fracture, and give an idea of the prognosis.
Photo: Dr. Ende

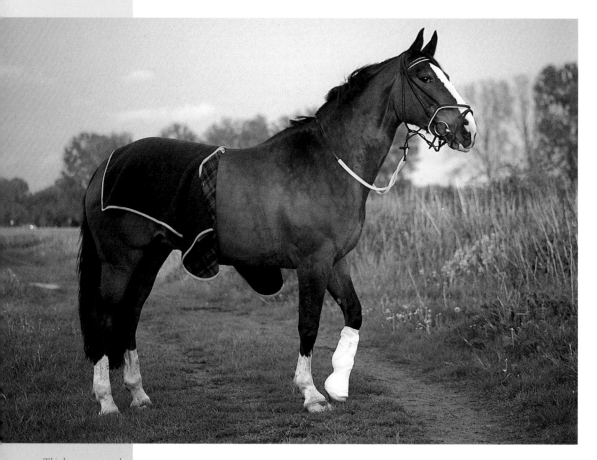

a displaced fracture. If you are there at the time, you will hear the break as a loud cracking noise. Once you have heard this sound, you will never forget it. With passive movement, displaced fractures will make a sound known as crepitation.

In almost every case, the bleeding will cause a fracture haematoma, a rapid, hot and painful swelling around the area of the fracture.

An X-ray is the only way to ascertain the nature and extent of a fracture. When you call the vet, you must tell him if you suspect a fracture, so that he can bring a portable X-ray machine. Open compound fractures, of course, are immediately

recognisable without X-ray. With closed fractures of the lower limbs and vertebral fractures, only an X-ray will be able to give a prognosis for healing.

Do not attempt to put a splint on or straighten out the fracture yourself. If you have to take the animal to a clinic, get a ready-made splint from your vet to stabilise the fracture. Splints using drainpiping or planks of wood should only be attempted if there really is no other way. Anything applied to the leg or bandages must be thickly padded.

With an open fracture, you should merely apply a clean, loose-fitting bandage and wait for the vet.

The transport of animals with broken limbs to be slaughtered is, in my opinion, unjustifiable.

Contrary to popular opinion, fractures are not only caused by traumatic events. Racehorses can suffer so-called fatigue fractures. Then there are fractures of the navicular or sesamoid bones, for example, which are preceded by chronic degenerative disease.

Young horses in good condition going on level ground can sometimes also experience fractures. The reason we always find this so hard to imagine is that, fortunately, it happens only rarely, and because we have no concept of the forces exerted by a horse placing a foot on the ground. In addition to the vertical force, there are significant tractive and gravitational forces which affect the bones.

I once had the pleasure of friendship with a four-year-old mare, apparently in perfect health, who very inconveniently managed to shatter her pastern bone on the lunge in the indoor school one Christmas Eve. Who knows, perhaps it was meant to be, but in those circumstances, what do you say to someone who wishes you a happy Christmas?

Unfortunately, fractures which happen while riding (trotting in the school or out on the gallops), leading in the yard, if the horse takes off in the jumping arena, or even in the stable, are a fact of life.

Fractures of the upper limb sections (forearm, point of shoulder) only occur as a result of significant trauma, such as a kick or a car accident.

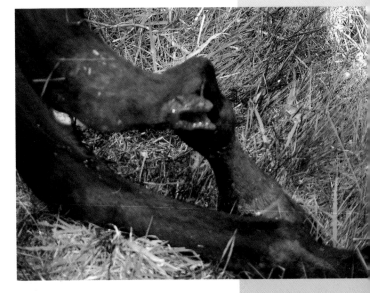

Compound fractures are still very often fatal.
Photo: Dr. Ende

Fractures of the pedal bone

The pedal bone is capable of breaking by itself, with or without the help of the hoof joint, or a sidebone which breaks.

Initially, no swelling can be seen. There is heat in the hoof wall and clear pulsation of the digital artery. The horse cannot put weight on the foot or is acutely lame. Where sidebones are broken, the symptoms are not quite so clear. X-rays from various angles will confirm the fracture.

Shortly after the fracture, the area above the hoof wall begins to swell.

Fractures of the pedal bone and the branch can heal conservatively, that is, without surgery.

Pedal bone fractures which enter the joint are unlikely to heal completely sound.

Fractures of the navicular bone

The navicular bone is a small boat-shaped bone which lies behind the pedal bone and is associated with navicular disease. In horses suffering from navicular disease, this bone degenerates to the extent that it can fracture. Sometimes, the middle of the bone dissolves and cysts are formed, which can lead to a fracture. There is considerable pain, although swelling is not noticeable at first. This bone does not have its own periosteum (it is a sesamoid) and regeneration is poor.

Great care must be taken with horses which have had a neurectomy as a result of navicular disease. The nerve leading to the toe has been surgically cut, and the horse no longer feels any pain in this area and, as a result, no longer protects the foot. Pressure is now being put on the already damaged bone, which does it no good at all, even if the horse feels no pain. At some point, it will simply break. Horses which have been de-nerved in this way should never jump. Regular (annual) X-ray checks should be made on the condition of the bone.

Fractures of the short pastern bone

Generally, the short pastern bone tends to shatter, and a joint is almost always involved. An operation can often be life-saving, but the prognosis for complete soundness is not good.

The horse will not put weight on the leg and significant swelling soon occurs above the hoof wall and in the pastern area.

Fractures of the long pastern bone

The long pastern bone can also shatter or break in a Y formation. The prognosis will depend on the involvement of the joint. An operation is available.

The horse will not put weight on the leg and significant swelling, which is very painful to the touch, soon occurs.

Fractures of the sesamoid bones

The sesamoid bones are the small triangular bones at the back of the fetlock joint. These bones do not have a periosteum and regeneration is poor. They are quite sensitive. The suspensory ligament is anchored at the top of these bones. With every step, very considerable forces are created in this area.

Sesamoid bones can break in two, or the tip can tear off.

These fractures can often be successfully operated on. Only an X-ray will provide clues to the extent of and prognosis for such fractures.

Fractures of the cannon bone

These fractures, too, are no longer necessarily fatal. Even compound fractures in this area can be successfully treated with surgery. Complete soundness is generally not achievable, but with patience on the part of horse and owner, and – of course – money, such fractures can heal perfectly well.

Fractures of the splint bones

Historically, splint bones are the remains of the second and fourth metatarsals. They start under the front knee joint or the hock and do not quite reach the pastern joint. Generally speaking, they are not required.

Fractures look and feel like splints. Horses with fractured splint bones can be lame. Very often, a great deal of new bone forms at the fracture point, forming a large lump which may press on important structures (such as the suspensory ligament). Sometimes, these fractures can be treated with special bandages, anti-inflammatory drugs and box rest, and only a lump will remain. Fractures which impede the horse's movement or will not heal with rest must be treated surgically. Usually, the splint bone above the over-reactive fracture point is severed and removed. Some protection will be needed after this, so that the bone stump does not proliferate. This type of fracture can cause problems if it is very close to the knee or hock.

Fractures in the knee and the hock

It is also possible for the many small bones which make up these joints to break. In the knee, fractures are usually the result of a fall or a kick. An X-ray will be required, and should be taken with the leg both standing and lifted.

Fractures of the forearm and second thigh

Fractures of the forearm are almost exclusively caused by a kick or in road traffic accidents. Most of these fractures are either compound or displaced. The horse is unable to put weight on the leg and the area around the fracture swells rapidly. Usually, this type of fracture will not heal, although on foals it can be treated with surgery.

Fractures of the second thigh require considerable force. Except in foals, they are almost always untreatable.

Fractures of the elbow

The majority of such fractures are the result of a kick. In a foal, it will usually heal, but in an older horse it will depend on the exact site of the fracture. Horses with such an injury will present with a very particular movement. Seen from the front, it looks as if the limb is being bent away from the body.

Fractures of the point of shoulder and the shoulder

Fractures of the point of shoulder and the shoulder are caused by falls. The horse will not bear weight and swelling can be clearly seen.

Fracture of the hip and pelvis

These, too, are primarily the result of falling. Fractures of the pelvis can often only be diagnosed by rectal examination, as X-rays are impossible on a standing, adult horse. Depending on the site and the effect on pelvic organs, fractures can heal with time.

Fractures of the cervical vertebrae

At the second cervical vertebra, fractures of the den, a process attaching to the first cervical vertebra, can occur. The horse will stand with its head and neck very stretched. Keep the horse calm and have an X-ray taken in the stable. Transport to the clinic may be an aggravation too far. With fractures of the cervical vertebra, it is absolutely essential to obtain a precise diagnosis from a vet and to follow his instructions to the letter.

Fractures of the spinous processes

Spinous processes occasionally break after a fall or an accident in the trailer. Very often, the horse will initially appear to be unhurt, but on the following day, his withers will be extremely sensitive to touch. Depending on the site and extent of the fracture, it will heal with or without surgery. However, it will take time (easily six months).

Fractures of the jaw

Fractures of the jaw can be caused by falling, getting caught by a guaranteed unbreakable headcollar, getting stuck in the bars of the stable, and biting on tying chains. They are easily recognisable because the jaw is easily accessible. In the lower jaw, only the sides can break. Unfortunately, however, they usually both break. In the upper jaw, one or several incisor teeth will usually break out upwards with or without part of the jawbone. This looks dramatic, but usually heals quickly and well with surgery.

10 Changes in the Stomach and Intestinal Tracts

Choking

Between the gullet and the stomach, a horse's oesophagus has three narrowings. Chewed food will pass through the first narrowing at the entrance to the rib-cage, the second above the heart and the third at the entrance to the stomach. Little bits of food can get stuck at all these points.

The classic causes of choking are sugar-beet shreds or pellets. Once it has become stuck, Ehis type of feed swells further, becomes harder and is less and less easy to dislodge. Other food particles might have been too large to start with and should not have been swallowed without being chewed.

If something does get stuck, the situation becomes dramatic for the horse. He will produce large amounts of saliva in an attempt to push the obstruction down. In doing so, he will lose fluid, which cannot be taken up by the intestine, since it will not

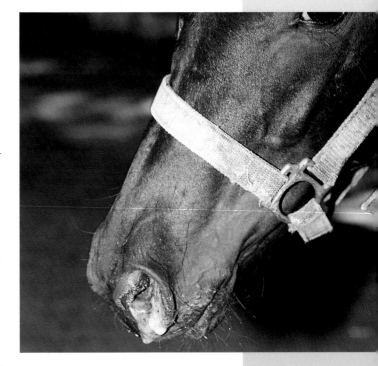

be able to reach that far. The loss of fluid visibly worsens the horse's general circulation. He will also panic, because he cannot breathe properly. We see such horses standing with

With choking, food particles may be found in the nasal discharge. Photo: Dr. Ende

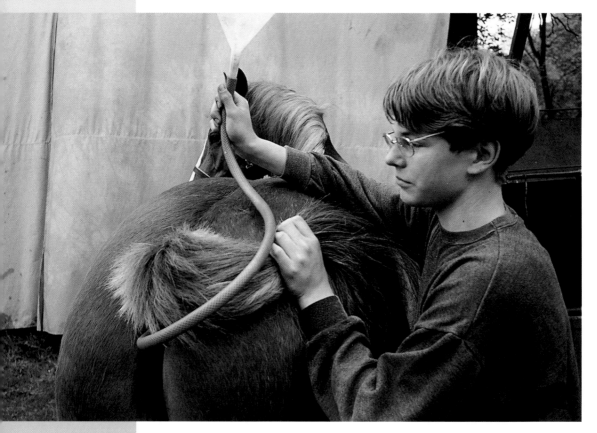

This is how to give an enema.
Photo: Dr. Ende

their necks stretched, and possibly also saliva and food particles in the nose.

The neck muscles may convulse. Body temperature will rise and the horse will not want to eat (although there are exceptions. I remember a little Welsh pony who began to choke one Sunday at a village fete, but was so unimpressed by his problem that he went on eating his hard feed until he could not possibly take any more in. We spent hours retrieving every tiny piece). If, in this situation, you ask the vet to come tomorrow, you will probably not need him at all.

Choking is a dire emergency, and can be fatal within hours if left untreated. While you wait for the vet, hold the horse's head low and, if you can feel the lump, massage it back towards the head. Offer water. Have buckets of warm and cold water ready. A towel would be nice, too.

With any luck, the horse will manage to swallow the lump by himself, but watch him for at least another couple of hours and only offer him water (no titbits – even if it is the right thing in virtually any other situation).

With a little less luck, the horse will be able to swallow the lump once the vet has given him a muscle-relaxing injection. Otherwise a nasal tube will have to be inserted to try to free the gullet and wash the obstruction down into the stomach. To do this, the vet will need to insert a plastic tube up the horse's nose and down into the oesophagus. A twitch will have to be applied. If the horse struggles, it may be that the ethmoid bone is broken. This causes profuse bleeding and can be frightening. If you are unable to bear it, go away and let someone else hold the horse.

In a few cases, it is not possible to deal with the problem in the stable and, in that event, your horse will need to be taken to the clinic as soon as possible. As a precaution, you could organise transport while you are waiting for the vet, then everyone will be relieved if the trip is unnecessary.

Think about what could have caused the choking, and tell the vet your suspicions.

If the obstruction has been cleared, the tube can be passed into the stomach and the typical smell of stomach acids will be noticeable at the end of the tube. It is better not to feed the horse for the rest of the day, and on the following day feed only hay. You can discuss with your vet whether you can feed anything else. You should keep a close eye on your horse for the next three days, and take his temperature every day. Following a choking episode, it is possible for lung infections to develop if the horse has breathed in food particles. Colitis, a resistant, evil-smelling scouring can also develop. Fortunately, this is rare in the stable. If it does arise, you will need to call the vet immediately.

Now that you know how choking can arise, you can try to prevent it.

Make sure that dry feed such as sugar-beet is adequately soaked before feeding. Make sure that horses have no access to the sugar-beet bin. Everything goes well for years, and then someone who doesn't know, or a child, comes along and feeds the "sweeties" to the horses. Never feed small apples or carrots (between 1.5 and 5cm diameter) whole. Do not give carrots sliced sideways. Carrot pieces become wedged into the narrowings of the gullet like a cork. If you must slice carrots, slice them lengthways. Whole garlic sections can also get stuck. If you chop up feed, either cut it so that the edges are less than a centimetre long or leave the pieces large enough so that they have to be chewed. Do not hand feed in situations where jealousy over food means that the horse would rather gulp the treat down whole.

Have your horse's teeth checked regularly by the vet (with annual vaccinations, for example). If your horse has a dental problem, or if he is old and his teeth are worn down, food should not be given in pieces.

Feed hay or soaked forage nuts, oats or mix to older horses, minerals in powder form and bananas. Everything else can be "pre-chewed" in a blender. All food must be freshly prepared!

Place "Please do not feed" signs on the fence and on the stable door – the best signs contain words and pictures. A carrot with a big cross through it cannot be misinterpreted, even by children or the illiterate.

If your field is next to houses, make a flyer which you can deliver to each house. Introduce yourself and your horses briefly, and list things that should not be fed and why (make sure you mention grass cuttings). Give a telephone number for people to contact if they have questions or so that they can report anything unusual in the field. This will create a neighbourly atmosphere, and will also benefit your horses.

Colic

Colic is the collective term for all painful processes in the abdominal area. Any colic attack can be life-threatening – call the vet!

You should suspect colic if your horse:

• won't eat
• lies down a lot
• has no stomach noises
• paws the ground
• looks at his abdomen
• looks as if he wants to stale
• kicks at his stomach
• adopts the flehmen posture
• rolls
• lies on his back while rolling
• "tucks up" his stomach muscles
• looks bloated
• has a high pulse rate
• sits like a dog.

Note: the above symptoms are never all present at the same time – just one will do for you to be suspicious!

Try to find out how your horse is. Is his circulation stable? Is there any audible stomach noise? Has he got a temperature? How clear are the signs of pain? When did he last eat, and what did he eat? Has he produced any droppings? When was the last

time? What did they look like? If possible, tell your vet the answers to all these questions on the telephone.

While waiting for the vet, walk your horse on a lead. If he doesn't want to walk, don't force him. If he wants to roll, let him. Offer him a little water. If he lies down, leave him for a maximum of five minutes, then ask him to walk a few steps before letting him lie down again.

If, should the need arise, you are prepared to let your horse undergo surgery for colic, make arrangements for transport to the veterinary clinic as a precaution. Longer-lasting episodes of colic can be kept under observation better in the clinic than at home in the stable. For one thing, the vet is on hand, and does not need to come back every two hours. Secondly, the laboratory can analyse a blood sample immediately, which is simply not possible when the vet is constantly on the move, and thirdly, at the clinic there will always be someone on duty at night.

Of course, you will need to choose a clinic which takes colic cases and which would be able to operate. It is arrant nonsense to take a horse to a general orthopaedic veterinary clinic, only to have to transfer him again if an operation becomes necessary. Your horse would certainly feel better at home. Discuss the sensible options for individual cases with your vet. If your horse has to go to the clinic, go with him. Stay by his side, but try not to get in the vet's way. By all means ask questions, but wait for an appropriate moment. When you get the all-clear after a few days, please remember, when you come to collect

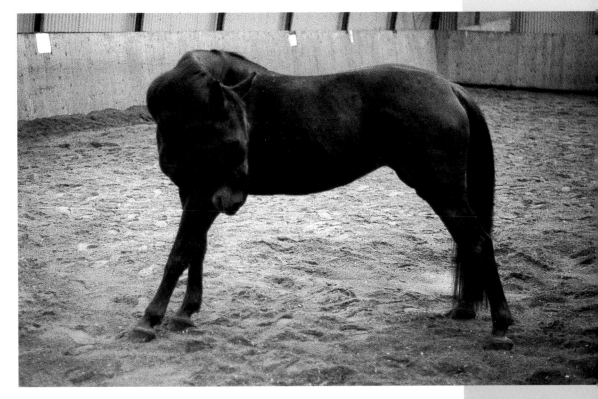

Clear symptoms of colic.
Photo: Dr. Ende

your horse, that the clinic's services may need to be paid for immediately.

However, say you are still at home with your sick horse waiting for the vet. What can you usefully do?

If you are able to, you can apply acupressure. The horse may find it comforting to have his abdomen massaged.

Covering with a rug or standing under a solarium can help horses whose circulation is stable.

Otherwise, the only advice is the advice which has been given for over a hundred years: lead the horse until the vet arrives.

If the horse stales, catch a small sample in a bucket.

Once the vet has arrived he will, as part of his investigations, have to carry out a rectal examination.

It is helpful if, in addition to the vet, two or three other people could be there to help (preferably competent young people or adults, not a gaggle of curious little girls who are complete novices with horses). One person should hold the horse's head, comfort it, and prevent it from rearing or running away. If necessary, the horse should be bitted or a twitch applied. At the moment, you only have the one vet there, and he is likely to suffer something of a sense of humour failure, not to mention a deterioration in his general health, if your horse kicks him. If you then compound the agony with statements such as "Did the naughty man hurt you, then?" or "Don't do that to the nice vet", don't be surprised if his reaction is somewhat chilly. If your horse rears during the examination, he could further injure his gut. This is a very bad thing, and should be avoided at all costs. If you have to let go of the horse during the examination, let him run forward rather than go up.

A second person should hold the tail up at the base, with all the hair out of the way. This will protect the vet from an angrily swishing tail and the horse from the small cuts which the tail-hairs can cause. If the horse clearly shows his displeasure at his treatment, it may be sensible to lift a foreleg. Wait for instructions to do this, but be available. If you have to tie up a hind leg, you will need a lunge line.

Other treatments can also be made easier by the presence of assistants, such as the insertion of a nasal tube, if the stomach has been overloaded and the horse is in pain, or intravenous injections, if the horse is badly behaved. Never forget how strong horses are. He is far more likely to be influenced by his painful gut than by the human hanging on his headcollar.

Colic can also be a slight cramp, which sometimes is weather-related, and which will have disappeared by the time the vet arrives. Be glad if this is what your horse's colic turns out to be, but don't just live in hope. Call the vet.

Colic pain is often also suffered by horses who have been out for too long on "good" or wet pasture. They tend to bloat, but there is usually a permanent improvement soon after the first injection.

Colics caused by impaction, twisting, invagination or displacement of the gut are usually associated with very painful clinical signs. Often, these cases can only be helped by surgery. Following the rectal examination, the vet will give you a diagnosis or a presumptive diagnosis, after which the decision will be whether or not to transport the horse to the clinic. If an operation is or may become necessary, transport should be sooner rather than later. This will significantly improve your horse's chances. These horses will often get better after the first injection, but will start to show symptoms again between thirty minutes and two hours later. This is when you go. If possible, get another pain-killing injection for the journey. Travelling in pain is unpleasant.

If your horse throws himself about in the trailer during the journey, don't panic. Whatever you do, do not open the front door of the trailer. If the trailer is closed, your horse will wedge himself into a position in which he is more comfortable (the crashing will then stop). Get a move on – things can't get much worse anyway. When you get to the clinic you and your horse will be helped. Equipment will be available to pull the horse out of the trailer if he has gone down. You cannot possibly do this by yourself somewhere along a country lane.

After the first injection, stay with your horse for at least two hours, and check him again after a further two hours. You can, of course, entrust this task to a reliable person.

Displacement of the intestine over the nephro-splenic ligament often results in minor colic symptoms, which come and go. A rectal examination will, however, produce a (presumptive) diagnosis. Often the gut sounds in the left upper quadrant are absent.

Obstructions build up slowly over a period of days. For example, if his fresh straw is really tasty, or if the horse is unaccustomed to it and – standing in the stable all day – eats it out of sheer boredom. On the day before, the droppings may be soft, since hard matter will already be unable to pass the obstruction. Obstructed in this way, the horse will be unable to dung or will only produce a few small dry droppings which will break on impact with the ground and are light brown or yellowish in colour. There are often no gut sounds in the lower intestinal region. Treatment can often extend over several days. Your horse will be put on a drip, and Glauber's salt in solution and oil will be given through a nasal tube. Your vet will need help and support. Whenever something in the gut finally gets moving, it will cause more pain. This is normal, but the horse may be better off at the veterinary clinic.

It is very dangerous to overload the stomach. Although horses have a fairly large intestinal tract, their stomachs are small. They can accommodate up to ten litres. This is not a great deal when you consider that not just food, but also saliva and the resulting gases that have to find space in there. Unfortunately, since

Outside, roughage can be offered in round bales. It would be better to feed it from a manger.
Photo: Dr. Ende

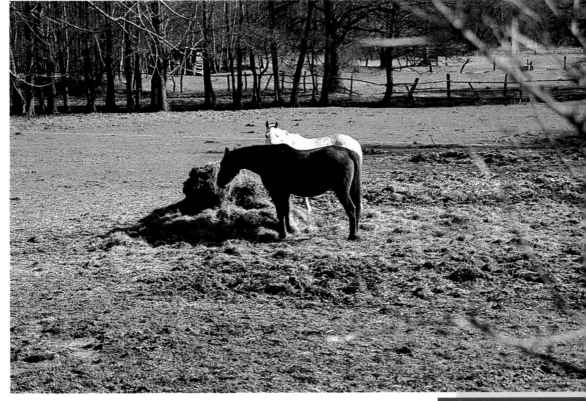

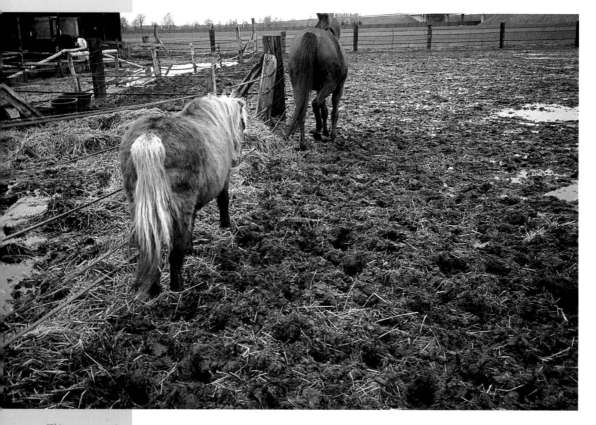

This arrangement is unhygienic and could easily lead to sand colic as well as to infected pasterns.
Photo: Dr. Ende

horses are unable to vomit, if the stomach becomes overfull even once, there is no relief.

Horses with an overloaded stomach will present with colic within one hour of eating. The symptoms are severe and the pulse rate is very high. The horse will sweat profusely at the neck. Time is of the essence, and a nasal tube needs to be inserted as a matter of urgency in order to provide relief before the stomach bursts.

Stomach overloads can also occur when the pulped food in the small intestine flows back into the stomach. You may need to transport the horse to the clinic with the nasal tube inserted by the vet still in place. The end of the tube should be fixed to the headcollar with adhesive tape.

Sand colic is the result of ingestion of sand or earth when a horse is in a paddock with little or no grass, or of eating unwashed root vegetables. The horse scours a little and only shows sporadic pain. It is possible that you will hear normal gut sounds from the lower stomach. Sand in the intestine sounds rather like waves running over a beach. Take one of your horse's droppings and dissolve it in a bucket of water. Stir it around well and swill out the bucket with a good swing. How much sand is left in the bottom of the bucket?

Heavy parasite burdens can trigger severe colic, which is difficult to treat. Tapeworms are also becoming more common. Consult your vet.

Colic pain can also be caused by

infections of the bladder or kidneys, bladderstones, displacement of the uterus and a number of other evils lurking in the horse's cavernous abdomen. Veterinary attention is absolutely essential for a diagnosis.

Try to prevent colic! Ultimately, of course, you will not be able to guarantee that it will never happen – after all, you are not a miracle worker. However, you can take the following precautions:

- Feed according to your horse's needs and in the correct sequence.
- Feed plenty of roughage before a meal (at least 1kg per 100kg of horse per day), followed by hard feed, if necessary. That way, the stomach will already be working when it has to deal with food which is harder to digest.
- Little and often is better than three large meals.
- Do not feed too much hard feed. These are horses, after all, not pigs to be fattened. Two kilograms per meal will suffice for a large horse.
- Introduce changes slowly, to allow the digestive bacteria to become accustomed to the differences.
- Prevent excessive eating of straw bedding.
- Do not allow the horse to drink large volumes after a feed.
- Have teeth checked regularly, and at least once a year.
- Keep parasites to a minimum through hygiene, good pasture management and regular worming.

If there are existing problems, there are a number of useful supplements which can help keep your horse's digestive processes in order:

- yoghurt
- yeast
- linseed (whole cooked linseed, not pre-prepared or mash)
- feed supplements with live yeast or lactic acids
- oil (small amounts of olive oil or – more cheaply – sunflower oil).

Scouring

Scouring should never be underestimated. It can be a symptom of a more serious underlying problem. The vet should be informed of any kind of scouring, but if it is runny and evil-smelling, call him immediately.

Isolate the horse (but so that he can still see his friends) and feed only clean water and good quality hay.

Never try to dry the scouring out by withdrawing the horse's access to water. You will probably only succeed in killing him.

Exceptions to this are suckling foals who are constant customers at mother's milk-bar. In these cases, you can and should prevent the excessive water intake.

Scouring in foals which occurs during the mare's foal-heat or as a result of infection with roundworms can also be dangerous. It is better to call the vet out once too often. Only conduct experiments after discussion with the vet. Withdrawal of fresh water and offering distilled water instead can be fatal. Human beings sometimes come up with very strange ideas.

Poisoning

First aid is not available for cases of poisoning. The horse is unable to vomit and what he has eaten will stay inside. Call the vet.

He will be able to administer substances which reduce absorption of the poison and expedite its passage through the intestine, so that it exits rapidly at the other end.

It is helpful if you can ascertain exactly what your horse has swallowed.

Some books describe the administration of coffee or anaesthetics, depending on the symptoms. Coffee can also be given directly into the intestine. These methods are old-fashioned and should only be applied in dire emergencies if you are unable to contact a vet, or if a vet has made a diagnosis and given you instructions to do so. At the end of the day, the nearest veterinary clinic won't be a million miles away. Until the vet arrives, offer the horse hay and water. You can then offer the coffee to the

Foxglove is pretty, but poisonous!
Photo: Dr.Ende

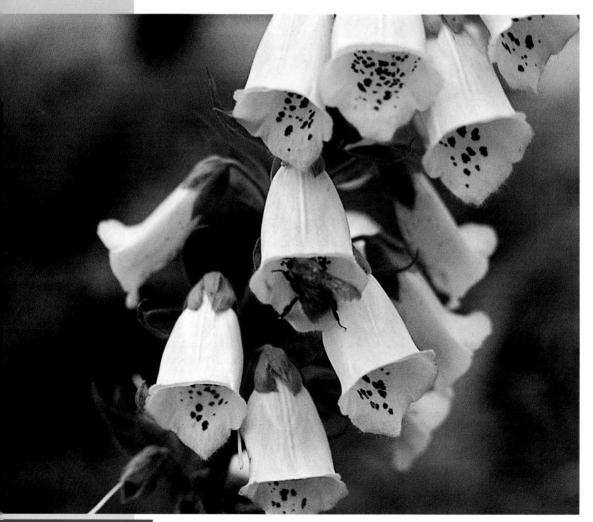

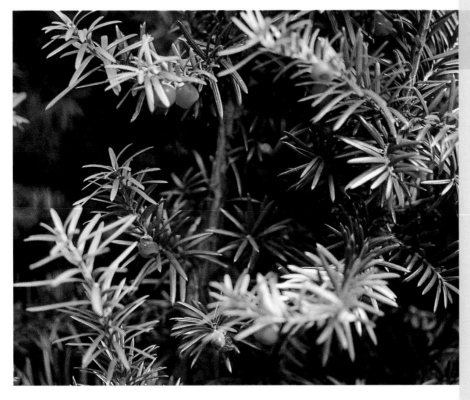

Yew is very poisonous.
Photo: Dr. Ende

vet when he arrives (he will drink it nicely out of a cup and will not require any tubes to be inserted).

The best thing you can do about poisoning is to prevent it. Ensure that nothing poisonous is growing in or immediately adjacent to the paddock. Horses who are used to living out will normally be able to distinguish between good and bad plants. If they are cut down, plants lose their typical appearance and horses will no longer recognise them. If the only bit of green the horse can reach from "fatty's paddock" is yew, he will probably eat it. Other tasty items (such as acorns) can be poisonous if eaten in excessive quantities.

Poisons can lurk in drinking water. If you are in doubt, have a sample tested.

Dead animals in the water tank can infect the whole system with botulism.

Meadow saffron in the hay is hard to spot, but is very poisonous.

Some mushrooms produce poisons which horses sometimes fail to recognise and eat.

When you are out riding, your horse may snatch at greenery at the side of the road. This is dangerous. He is, after all, only interested in taking advantage of your momentary lack of attention and will not make a careful assessment of what he is eating.

It can also be dangerous to take the horse home and let it have a browse through the garden. There may be plants which he doesn't know (lily of the valley, potato, tulips...) but may be curious about, like the strange foods (for example kiwi fruit, oranges or bananas) he sometimes takes from your hand.

Horses can sometimes be unwittingly poisoned by neighbours. Explain to neighbours what horses can and can't eat, otherwise you will constantly find cabbages and potato peelings in your field, as well as mouldy bread, vegetable waste and grass cuttings. In this case, good intentions are just the opposite.

You and the young people in your yard can learn a lot about poisonous plants. Books on poisonous plants and other aspects of equine welfare are available from the BHS.

Learning can be fun, and Pony Club rallies can incorporate questions about poisonous plants into their games.

11 Azoturia

Sometimes referred to as tying up, Monday morning disease, haematuria or lumbago, azoturia is an acute affliction of the muscles of the hindquarters. It comes on suddenly, looks awful, is very painful for the horse and must be treated immediately.

During or after work, the horse will suddenly become shaky or lame behind or may not move at all. The muscles of the hindquarters become rock hard and are very painful. The pulse rate and temperature rise. You can see by the horse's expression that he is in severe pain. It appears as if his eyes are about to pop out of their sockets. He may also sweat profusely.

Dismount immediately and do not move the horse – at all. If you are out on a hack, you can travel the horse home. Call the vet immediately. While you wait for him to arrive, you can lightly cover the horse's back with a rug.

These symptoms always appear after unusually hard work. Another trigger is usually work which follows a rest day with too much food. "Too much food" and "unusually hard work" are relative terms. Full rations with no work is always too much, and work which follows a rest day should always be careful. In that sense, a gallop around the field on a rest day can already be unusually hard work for an unfit horse.

If he is built up by regular work and correct feeding, no horse should experience azoturia.

12 Laminitis

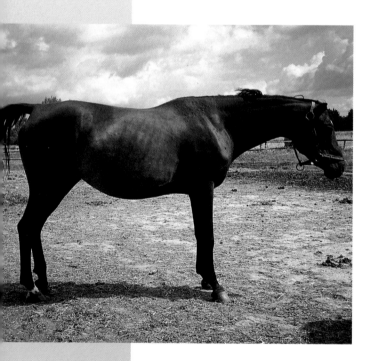

This stance is typical of laminitis.
Photo: Dr. Ende

laminitis is an intake of too much fresh spring grass, but too much hard feed, hard work, infections, poisoning and retention of the placenta after foaling are some of the other causes. The initial signs are a pottery gait, pulsation of the arteries at the fetlock and warming of the hooves. Laminitis can occur in just one foot, just the front feet or in all four feet. If you suspect laminitis, call your vet and your farrier. Put your horse on a strict diet of old hay and water straight away and cool the affected feet. If it is not laminitis, you will not do any harm. If it is laminitis, this is the only way in which you can have some influence on the progress of this painful and dangerous condition.

Laminitis is always an emergency. Anything you fail to do within the first twelve hours cannot be put right afterwards. Amongst other causes of

13 Tetanus

Tetanus or "lockjaw" is a life-threatening condition with a dramatic phenotype. Initially, a horse suffering from tetanus will become stiff and disinclined to move, and this stiffness will spread until the neck becomes stiff and the face looks very tense. The third eyelid may appear in the corner of the eye and looks like a piece of skin travelling across the eye. Finally, the horse will stand with his legs splayed out and will not move. He may also be cast. At this stage it is usually too late. If you have early suspicions of tetanus, call the vet and tell him what you suspect.

Take the horse into a darkened, quiet stable. There must, of course, have been some injury for the condition to be triggered, but it may have been very minor and overlooked.

Tetanus symptoms take days, sometimes even weeks, to develop, by which time the original wound has completely healed. Fortunately, you and your horse will never encounter this problem, because you will have ensured that his tetanus vaccinations are always up to date.

In the book-world, there is a publication the author of which recommends that vaccination be dispensed with and states that horses develop their own natural immunity to tetanus. Clearly, they do not all succeed in doing so, since a number of horses still die a horrible death from the condition. Anyone who has ever seen the suffering of a horse with tetanus will never again do without this inexpensive and well tolerated solution.

14 Shock

In an emergency, your horse may go into shock. This can happen in an accident, in a fire, with colic, scouring, heavy bleeding, poisoning, casting or heatstroke.

You will hardly be able to feel a pulse, which will have a rate of eighty to one hundred beats per minute. Skin elasticity is disrupted and a pinched fold of skin will initially not return to its normal state. Capillary filling time will be increased. The horse will be apathetic and will not react to stimulants such as your voice – whether you talk to or shout at him – or touch. He may start to shiver.

Stabilising infusions are urgently needed. If a vet doesn't arrive very quickly, you can still help your horse. Prepare a salt solution (100g of ordinary cooking salt to 10 litres of water) warmed to body temperature. Insert a plastic hosepipe – on which you will have rounded and greased the ends – gently into the rectum so that it reaches approximately 15cm into the intestine, and pour in the salt solution using a funnel.

As described in the chapter which deals with fire (chapter 18), you can also give oxygen.

Rescue remedy drops are not wrong, either.

15 Heatstroke

Horses are relatively impervious to heat, although they can sometimes become overheated if left out in blazing sunshine.

It is particularly dangerous if the horse becomes excited and makes demands on its own system without taking in sufficient water or pausing to rest in the shade. It is irresponsible of us to ask our horses to work in the heat without offering them water and appropriate rest breaks.

In an overheated horse, the rectal temperature can reach 43°C. The horse will stagger and break down, shiver, become unaware of his surroundings and register very high pulse and respiratory rates. He will be in urgent need of an infusion from the vet.

Splash cold water over the horse's legs and bring him into the shade. Cover him with damp cloths (replace them when they dry out). If he is unable to walk to the nearest shady area, try to make a sun-shield for him. Offer him water. As with shock, you can given him a salt water infusion.

Prevention is better than cure: make sure that your horses have some sort of shelter out of doors. This can be in the form of an open stable, a field shelter, a Dutch barn or a clump of large, old trees. Do not make too many demands of even otherwise robust horses.

Ensure that fresh water is always available in sufficient quantities. Three inches of green slime at the bottom of the tank is not enough. Defective automatic drinkers and fillers must be repaired in order to avoid horses dehydrating.

If you ride in warm or hot weather, do not ask too much of your horse. Have breaks and, on longer rides, offer him water. Get your horse used to drinking out of containers other than his own bucket.

If you are out on a very long ride, stop to measure pulse and respiratory rates and pinch the skin to test its elasticity.

16 Urticaria

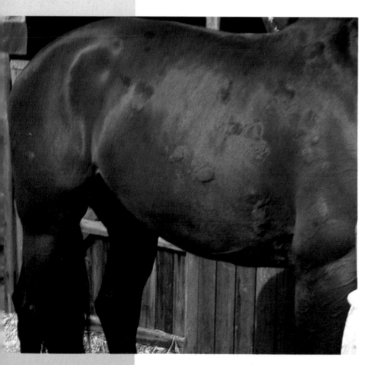

This horse is covered with nettle rash. This is an allergic reaction.
Photo: Dr. Ende

Urticaria is caused by contact with or ingestion of substances which cause an allergic reaction (allergens). The horse becomes restless, tries to roll and will rub himself on anything which appears to him to be appropriate. Within minutes, he will be covered with hives, which can range from the size of a pinhead to the size of a £2 coin. His breathing may be stertorous, and his pulse rate and body temperature will rise. Left untreated, the condition can develop into shock and can be life-threatening. In some horses, the head swells to such an extent that your previously elegant horse now looks like a hippopotamus. The mucous membranes in the nose and throat can also swell, which makes breathing extremely difficult. The horse will not want to be touched. The cause of the outbreak should be removed. If you see a reaction like this following an insect bite or following application of a medicine or after food, there will not be a great deal you can do. However, if the horse has reacted to a new fly repellent, hose the horse down. Water and cold towels can relieve the symptoms until the vet arrives. Keep an eye on the horse's circulation.

17 Foaling

If you are planning to breed from your mare, think it through thoroughly before you start.

You should only breed from your mare if you are prepared to keep the foal. If you have to sell it, it will break your heart. Part of your responsibility is to be able to offer the foal a future. There are already far too many horses, even good ones, facing an uncertain future. The sale rings are full of potential hopefuls who don't even cover their costs. Breeding is not a good source of income.

Make sure you use only a healthy mare and choose an appropriate stallion. Take advice – but not from the owner of the stallion.

Take into account the costs in time and money, and consider whether you really want to take on the difficulties associated with the whole process.

Consider whether you are in a position to offer the pregnant mare – and later the foal – ideal conditions.

The expense begins prior to covering. Give your mare supplements containing carotene and have swabs taken. If the mare is clean, have her hind shoes removed and take her to the stallion.

Scans for pregnancy can be taken at 18, 40 and 120 days.

Continue to ride the mare and don't overfeed her. Do not give any drugs, even wormers, during the first trimester of pregnancy.

Have the mare vaccinated against virus abortion and tetanus.

Worm the mare once more before foaling; there will be fever worms in the mare's milk and the foal will carry less of a burden.

Move the mare into the foaling box in good time. The box should have been thoroughly cleaned. Muck out daily and make banks of straw.

Accustom the mare to having her teats handled and keep them clean. Also accustom her to the emergency night-time lighting. If you do not

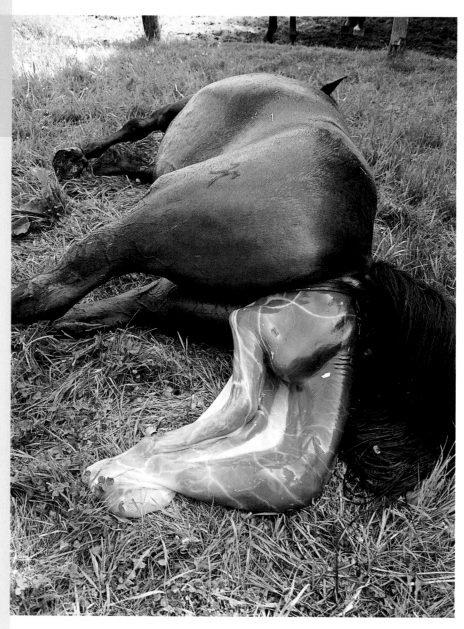

Foaling in the open is
natural and, if the
weather is good,
problem-free. However,
it is harder to
supervise.
Photo: Dr. Ende

think you can deal with it, let the mare foal at an animal clinic. In principle, you need do nothing about the actual foaling, because the mare can manage much better by herself. Otherwise, you will need transport if a caesarean section becomes necessary. If you need the vet, you will need a telephone. If you want to help the mare yourself, you will need sterile single-wear gloves.

In the early stages, you need only to keep watch. If anything appears abnormal, call the vet.

Once the waters have broken, the amniotic sac will appear at the vulva.

The sac will contain both forefeet with the soles level and facing downwards. The head will be lying on the pasterns. Normally, the foal will then be expelled quickly by the contractions. As long as the umbilical cord remains intact, the foal will be fed by the mare. If the birth canal is very narrow, the foal may become wedged. At this point, you can (with your gloved hands) carefully grasp the pasterns and pull. Pull only if the foal appears to be lying in the correct position, and only during a contraction. Once the foal has arrived, you can make a tear in the foetal membrane, if it is still unbroken, and free the nose. If the foal does not start to breathe by itself, massage the ribcage with straw. Leave the umbilical cord alone: it will break by itself in the proper place. You can then dip the end which remains hanging from the foal in iodine solution. Once this is done, leave the box and return quietly to your observation post.

The foal should be standing within one hour. After two hours it should be searching for the mare's teats and suckling. After those two hours, the placenta should also have been delivered. If the placenta is hanging out, do not pull at it. If there is a risk of the mare treading on it, tie it up. Do not tire the foal. If the mare is badly torn, bleeding heavily or if the placenta has not been pushed out after two hours, call the vet. Also call him if the placenta is incomplete, or if the foal is not standing and suckling in good time, even in the middle of the night. It's important.

Check whether the foal has passed urine and droppings. If it has not done so in the first twelve hours, you will need the vet. A prophylactic antibiotic injection – in combination with vitamins – is available against paralysis in new-born foals, for which you may need him on the morning after the birth in any event.

18 Burns

Everybody's worst nightmare: the stables are on fire!

Call the fire brigade immediately and – only provided it appears reasonably safe for you to do so – try to get the horses out as quickly as possible. The horses will be absolutely terrified, having difficulty breathing because of the smoke and may already have suffered burns. This is the first time they will have ever experienced anything like this and they will not understand what is happening. We have always taught them that their stable is their refuge. This notion will now have to be actively reversed.

You will have to convince them that "It's nothing to worry about". Put the horse's headcollar on as normal and quietly lead the horse out of the stable on a lead rope. Do not go into the stable alone. If the horse will not follow, cover his eyes with a cloth and a second person can push from behind. Do not shout at or hit him.

He will be frightened enough already.

For as long as you are trying to get the horses out alive, keep windows shut. Use the first of any available water to make yourself wet. You can be a hero, but you must make the distinction between caution and cowardice, courage and recklessness.

If you have succeeded in getting the horses out, do not simply leave them just outside the stable – hand them over to helpers or take them into a secure paddock.

Watch out for signs of shock. The horse's airways may have been damaged by smoke. The mucous membranes will be blue in colour. If the horse is lying down and showing clear symptoms of shock you can, while you are waiting for the vet to arrive or until you have to leave for the clinic, pump up to 15 litres of oxygen into the horse's nostrils using an oxygen bottle, which you can obtain from a metal works, and a small tube. Otherwise, the horse will be considerably helped by the fresh air outside. Offer water as soon as possible. Burns must be kept very clean.

The best coverings are cloths which have been ironed and dipped in clean water or mild salt solution.

Horses which have been rescued from burning stables will be intensive care patients for several days afterwards. They will be vulnerable to infections of their lungs and airways, liver damage and all sorts of other infections, as well as having large wounds which do not heal well.

It is best if they can spend this time in a veterinary clinic.

Of course, it would be even better if there had been no fire. For the sake of your own and your horse's welfare, and to avoid subsequent aggravation with insurance companies, take precautions and fit smoke alarms. In larger yards, it would be sensible to have fire drills and develop contact with your local fire services.

Fire extinguishers should be available in sufficient numbers. They should also be in working order, and therefore need regular testing. A hydrant or emergency water supply must be available and in working condition.

Hay and straw should not be stored immediately adjacent to the stables. Smoking should never be allowed on the yard. The same applies to naked flames. Bonfire night can be celebrated elsewhere, even if there is a lot of combustible rubbish on the yard.

Open fires must be supervised. A strong wind is the worst possible weather in which to make a fire. Check and maintain electrical installations and equipment regularly.

Yards and stables should not be locked. If they have to be locked for security reasons, there must be a central unit from which they can all be unlocked at once. If there is a fire, no-one has time to unlock each individual stable. Apart from that, the locks will be getting hot.

It is sensible to install smoke alarms in the barn or in the hayloft. It might also be an idea to enquire about installing a lightning conductor. If you decide to do so, have it regularly maintained. Defective lightning conductors attract lightning!

Hay and straw should be stored dry, otherwise there is a risk of spontaneous combustion.

Everybody must be aware of the risks. Regular fire drills can raise risk awareness. Children should know that matches, lighters, glass and mirrors have no place in the barn.

Catalytic converters can get very hot, so cars should not be parked on the dry grass behind the stables.

You have thought of everything. Unfortunately, the old kettle in the shed short-circuits …

Make a game of it. Every participant has one week in which to compile a list of all the risks he comes across and how they could be reduced. Whoever finds the most sources of danger is the winner.

19 Horse Transport

Always consider whether a journey is really necessary. If you are involved in an accident en route, it will be all the more annoying if you only went to do someone else a favour, and neither you nor your horse had any real interest in the outing.

If you do want to make a journey, plan it well in advance. If you regularly travel to competitions with your own trailer you will, of course, need to do this less than if you only travel occasionally with borrowed equipment.

Horses can be transported in trailers, lorries, by air or sea, depending on the nature of the journey and your own resources. A trailer is the usual form of transport for shorter routes with one horse. If you have your own trailer, ensure that it is roadworthy, and that the floor, partition and bolts are in good condition. If you plan to purchase a trailer, get all the information you possibly can. Prices and equipment vary significantly. Safety standards are far higher now than they were even a few years ago.

If you intend to borrow a trailer, check it over thoroughly. Even vehicles hired out by commercial firms are not always guaranteed to be roadworthy.

You can choose between a single or double trailer, and a tarpaulin or plastic roof. The latter looks much better, but if there is no ventilation, after a two-hour traffic jam on a summer journey, the horses will be cooked through.

Inspect the floor. Pick up the rubber matting and look for rotten or badly sealed areas. All the bolts should be intact and all the lights in working order. Test the suspension. Brakes? Is the transmission cable the right one for your vehicle?

Choose a trailer from which the front bars can be removed from outside.

The towing vehicle must be well able to cope with the weight it will

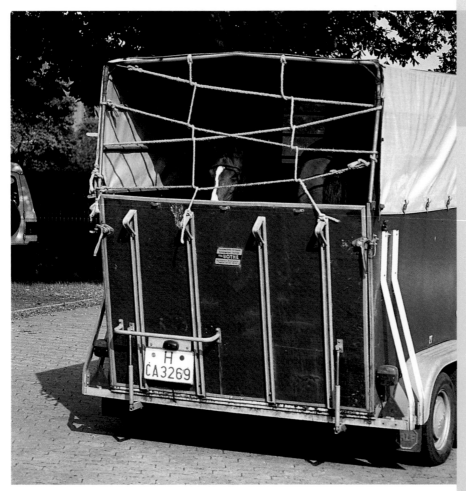

be required to pull. If you are borrowing the towing vehicle as well, check it over. Fill the tank when the trailer is not attached.

Towing needs practice. You owe this to your horse. A number of companies offer free training on their own premises and at trade fairs.

Practise loading your horse. He should follow you into the trailer quickly and willingly. If necessary, get help from someone with experience. Make sure the trailer is suitable for your horse. You may need a second front bar or a panel to prevent

ponies and smaller horses from ducking underneath. You can also do entirely without a partition or front bars.

If you are towing foals or Shetland ponies that are not tied up, or if you are towing on the motorway, close the top door panels.

When you are travelling, never open the front ramp if you are not sure that your horse is standing behind it.

Give yourself plenty of time for loading and travelling. If you possibly can do not travel in the middle of

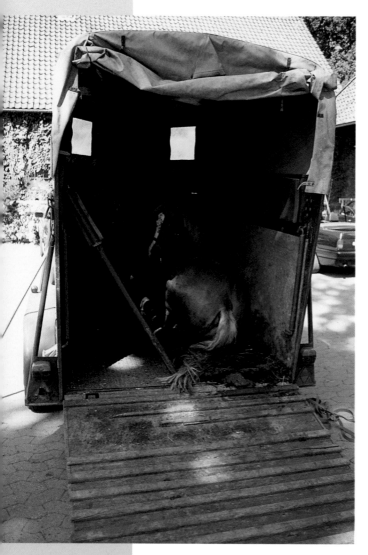

This kind of accident in a trailer is amongst the most dangerous and the most dramatic.
Photo: Dr. Ende

supervise. I am, of course, perfectly well aware that this is not common practice at showgrounds, either with trailers or lorries. It is important, however, since a horse who suddenly feels the want of some company can do himself severe damage in an open trailer. You will probably also have difficulties with the insurance company.

If you drive a lorry, check the wheelnuts regularly, and then again between inspections.

If you like, your horse can be transported by a commercial transporter. These come in all shapes and sizes. Big, not quite sober men who usually transport pigs but are willing to give it a go with a horse. Might be friendly and certainly cheap, but are they really suitable? Ask around whether anyone knows a good transporter. There are companies (although I'm not allowed to advertise them here) who can transport horses better and more comfortably than we can ourselves.

Transport by ship means that you can accompany your horse, although you may have to ask about this. He will enjoy travelling with his own personal steward. It is also a good way of ensuring that no-one abuses him and that he is regularly fed and watered.

Generally speaking, you will not be able to accompany your horse on an aeroplane journey, although you can accompany him as far as the container in which he will travel. These days, such containers are very comfortable. For safety reasons, the transporter will appoint a qualified person to accompany you both.

the day during the summer. Do not drive too fast. Tie your horse up short in the trailer and use a well-fitting headcollar and a leadrope which is in good condition. Your horse should have at least his forelegs protected by bandages or travelling boots, which must reach over the heel.

If you are transporting more than one horse, unload them one by one. If one horse has to wait in the trailer, someone should stay with him to

All this is self-evident, everybody knows it; but accidents continue to happen, lots of accidents. Almost all of them are unnecessary and avoidable.

If your horse is rampaging in the trailer, pull over and go and see what the trouble is from the back – do not open the front ramp.

If he has fallen, you will have to get him up again. If the trailer is closed, drive to a place where doing so will not interfere with the traffic or be dangerous for your horse. Sometimes it is possible to move the bars sufficiently from outside the trailer for the horse to be able to get up by himself once he has been pulled back a bit.

It is really dangerous if any part of your horse has left the trailer. Either a foot through the floorboards, or a leg appearing through the groom's door, which has unfortunately come open. Stop the vehicle and trailer immediately (gently) and try to push the leg back into the trailer. Only then can you get the horse out of the back of the trailer, or pull him if he has fallen down. In modern trailers, you can release the bars from outside. On the outside at the front of the trailer are tying rings which can be turned. In older tarpaulin-topped trailers, these can be cut open and the bars dismantled from there. If the horse is not lying too awkwardly, treatment for shock and, if necessary, sedatives can be administered by the vet in the trailer.

If you are unable to rescue your horse yourself, call the fire brigade. If you are obstructing the highway, you will also need to notify the police. If your trailer has overturned, it is best to right it again before releasing the horses. If there is only one horse, the trailer can be cut open while it is lying on its side.

Accidents with trailers sometimes involve serious and occasionally untreatable injuries. Once you have seen a few such accidents, you can only stand and stare in disbelief at some of the trailers and conditions in which horses are expected to travel.

A leg which has gone through the floorboards and been dragged along a tarmac road at speed will be sliced off – shoe, hoof, skin and pedal bone will be gone. What help do you give in such situations?

Loose partitions which buckle when leaned on will require highly experienced and careful horses if you want to reach your destination in one piece. It is unreasonable to expect your horse to deal with bars which are not fixed, or fixed temporarily with pipe cleaners because the ring fell off weeks ago. Sadly, it often takes something serious to happen before these things are given any real thought.

If you buy or sell a horse which will be transported to its new home, be very clear as to who owns the horse while it is travelling. If the change of ownership takes place before the journey, the new owner should have insured the horse for third party liability before the journey.

If someone does you a favour, enquire about the insurance position. If you transport someone else's horse as a favour, and the horse is injured en route, either because of your driving style or because the trailer is defective, you will be paying for the favour for a long time if you have no written agreement. If your trailer is wrecked, you will probably have to pay for its replacement yourself. If you lend someone your trailer in return for a consideration, make sure you have a written agreement.

This is not as far-fetched as it sounds. Here are two examples:

A person goes on holiday with two horses, which travel in a trailer borrowed from a riding instructor friend free of charge. Even before they reach the motorway, the floor of the trailer gives way and a foot goes through. The horse's injuries are not life-threatening, but still bad enough. The trailer is a write-off. The owner of the horses is in shock. The accident happened on a main road and the police were involved. The trailer turned out to be unroadworthy. The aggravation which can arise out of such situations is not inconsiderable.

Someone buys a horse. The horse is to travel to the purchaser's home some 25km away. A friend of the seller transports the horse with her car and a borrowed trailer. Both the seller and the buyer are present during the journey. Two kilometres from their destination, the groom's door opens, perhaps because the horse kicked at it. The horse loses his balance and falls down. The accident happens at night at a busy junction. The police, fire brigade, vet and helpers turn out. The trailer is very badly damaged, but the horse is rescued with relatively minor injuries. In this situation, who is responsible for what? Was the horse, which is now sadly injured, already sold, or did he still belong to his previous owner? If everything had gone well, the question would never have arisen. It would have been better, though, to have clarified the situation beforehand.

20 Casting

Horses can get themselves into the most impossible situations. If you find a horse in a situation from which he cannot free himself, talk to him, so that he knows you are there, and then consider what to do next. If you need the vet and the fire brigade, call them. Do not put yourself in danger.

Casting in the stable

Do not open the stable door. If you do, a head, legs or other parts of the horse could fall out and cause serious injury, because the horse will immediately try to free himself. Also, you will be unable to shut the door again once you have realised your mistake. So – the door stays shut.

In order to be able to get up, the horse will need space in front of him, and will need to bring his hind legs underneath him. If the situation doesn't look too impossible, try to persuade the horse to make another attempt to get up by himself. Sometimes, they do just need convincing.

If that doesn't work, and the horse's legs are up against the wall, you will have to help him by turning him over. This is perfectly possible, even for a small-framed woman. Technique is everything. Using lunge lines, you will need to make a loop around the pasterns of the lower legs. Try not to get kicked. This is the most difficult part. Take the other end of the lunge lines into the next-door stable or over the stable door – depending on where the horse is lying. If you have to go into the next-door box, tie the occupant up or ask someone to hold him. Do not take him away. He will be out of the way, but if you take him right away the cast horse may panic. Do not help the cast horse to turn over while you are still in the stable with him. For some horses, the joy of sudden freedom makes them react over-

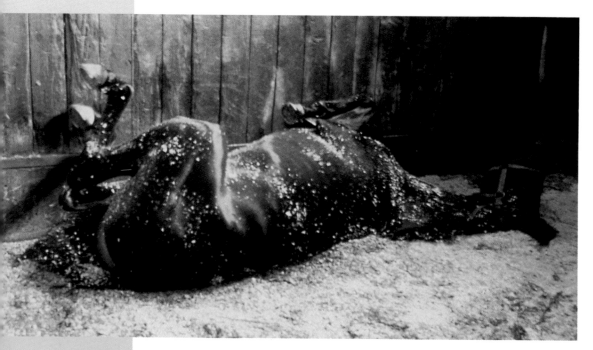

This horse will be unable to get up without help. If he is turned over on his back, he will be able to get up without difficulty.
Photo: Dr. Ende

enthusiastically. Pull the horse over on its back using the lunge lines. If he stays down, encourage him to get up with your voice or tickle him with the end of a schooling whip. Enter the stable only once the horse is standing, remove the lunge lines and walk the horse out in hand for a few minutes. Trot him up to check for lameness, inspect his head and legs for injuries and treat any you find. Check his eyes for injuries, too.

If the horse is lying with his head and chest close to a wall or in a corner, it really only needs to be pulled back a bit. However, this is too hard for one person alone, and too dangerous, because you will be in the stable throughout the process. With at least one other assistant, grasp the dock of the tail, the mane and the headcollar and pull. If the distance between the bars or boards of the stable is more than one hoof's width,

it may be that a leg has become jammed between them. If you find the horse too late, it may be that he has broken a hip or is already dead. If he is still alive, he probably fell down while trying to free himself. Free him by breaking the bars. You should, of course, talk calmly and quietly to him while saws and crowbars are being used. Once you have released the horse, leave him lying down. He will be exhausted. If he tries to get up by himself, you can support him by holding the headcollar and the dock. Only once he is standing can you make a proper assessment of the damage.

Always make sure that the dimensions and construction of any stable are suitable for the horse that is to occupy it, particularly with smaller horses, ponies, young horses and stallions. If neighbours kick at one another, a leg can easily become wedged in the bars. Many horses can kick above their own height with their back legs.

Always check to see why the horse became cast. Did he have stomach-ache and roll? If so, he may well still have stomach-ache and this should be investigated. Horses will also roll because of skin allergies, uncomfortably matted hair or simply for pleasure. Also check him the next day for crush injuries, bruises and lameness.

Casting in the stable is, although not always, becoming easier to prevent. Choose a stable that is large enough for your horse. Some particularly clumsy individuals can get themselves cast against a fence in the field. Install mangers and automatic drinkers in such a way that they do not become horse-traps. Bank up the bedding along the sides of the stable, so that the horse will tend to lie in the middle of the stable rather than against the sides. Avoid deep litter. In the struggle to free himself, there is a risk that he will shovel mountains of old bedding under his legs, and getting up will become harder and harder. Ensure that the floor is not slippery, even if it is wet (if need be, use peat as a base). If your horse still insists on getting himself cast, buy him an anti-cast roller, which will allow him to lie down and walk about, but will stop him rolling right over on his back. Allow your horse the time and the pleasure of rolling regularly in an appropriate spot (field, paddock, school). Do not leave the horse in the stable if he is wet or muddy. Hose him down or brush him.

Casting outside

Both in and out of doors, horses will only be able to free themselves if they have space in front of them and are able to get their hind legs underneath them. Occasionally, it will be possible to pull the front legs forward with lunge lines. Try to keep the head forwards and up.

In the field, horses can become cast under fences or in ditches. They can often be pulled out from under fences. If they are caught up in the fence, you will have to turn the power off, and you may need your wire cutters. For a horse stuck in a ditch, you will normally need specialised equipment. Call the fire brigade. You must keep calm, both while waiting for the fire brigade to arrive and during the rescue operation. Try to remove any pieces of fence, gate or whatever else went into the ditch together with your horse. If you can, put a sturdy headcollar on. If need be, hold his head up so that he can breathe more easily. If you can reach him without falling into the ditch yourself, you can put some rescue remedy drops inside his bottom lip. Look out for signs of shock.

Horses can become stuck in ponds with soft banks or marshes.

It will be necessary to attach straps around his chest and abdomen by which he can be pulled out. If the saddle and girth are still in place, the girth can be used as a guide for the straps, so do not remove his tack immediately. Try to prevent the horse from struggling. While you are waiting for help to arrive, you may be able to get an old tree branch, tyre or similar solid object which may be lying around under him for support and to prevent him from sinking further. Do not put yourself in danger.

Falling through thin ice

If your horse falls through thin ice, try to motivate him to head for the bank. Hold his head at a distance. You could try to ride him out, which is unpleasant, but less risky than being next to him.

It is rare that a horse will fall into a swimming pool or a quarry pool. It is possible for them become trapped under ice. With the help of the fire brigade, and by using your knowledge of horses and plain common sense, you will have to find individual solutions for rescuing your horse from such situations. The vet may need to anaesthetise the horse.

This type of accident usually only happens if horses are unsupervised or are able to get out of their field. The unscheduled separation of horse and rider can also be a cause of sheer panic, which will only be increased if other objects such as the cart, the shafts, or the fence to which it was tied are also attached to the horse.

Again, the only really good advice is prevention.

Place fences at some distance from ditches. If the horse puts its head under the fence to graze, he can easily lose his balance. When chased by other horses, a horse can suddenly and temporarily develop an amazing talent for jumping (even horses who, with a rider on board, would refuse cavaletti). There must either be enough room to land behind the fence or a sizeable object that would stop the horse from attempting to jump out, such as a hedge or a wall. A ditch does not constitute such an object, because the horse will only see it as he is falling into it.

Ensure that all the places where your horse goes are secure. Going exploring on his own is simply not allowed, however authoritarian that sounds.

Always ride on designated bridleways. If you practise going through water, do not do so alone or in out-of-the-way places. Do not experiment. It is not boring and uncool to turn around and meet the challenge better equipped next time, it is responsible and safe.

21 The Hardest Choice

There are times when treatment is possible, but not sensible. Sometimes, death is the more "humane" solution. Think about this in a situation in which you are not affected. Would you, if it became necessary, allow your horse to undergo an operation for colic? This type of decision often means weighing up the balance between a number of evils.

It may well be right to do everything to sustain life in every case. What happens, however, if there are sequels which mean that you and your horse will have to endure a lifetime of problems, to which there may, in the end, be no solution? This raises the question of what we can, and should, reasonably expect of our horses, how much we are able and prepared to invest in terms of time and effort, and how much we are prepared to do without. And, lastly but by no means least, what we can afford financially.

Please do not think that your own solution is the only right one. If someone in your immediate vicinity has decided against treatment and opts for euthanasia, do not be critical. The decision is hard enough, and cannot be undone afterwards. Even if you think "perhaps you could have ...", your criticism is of little use after the event. If you think, however, that someone is "loving their horse too long" and is perhaps even being cruel because they are too fearful of making the final decision, talk to them, but try to see the situation from their point of view, and don't make the decision for them.

Discuss this question with others. Individually, you can seek advice from your vet.

Unfortunately, the word "impossible" is part of our language. Some situations arise in which the horse simply cannot be helped and must be put to sleep. If it can be done swiftly and painlessly, so much the better.

There is always the comfort of knowing that he is no longer suffering.

Horses can be put down by means of a humane killer or by lethal injection.

The one is no worse than the other. In the cases we are talking about here, it will be a release in any event. If you have your horse put to sleep by injection, you or someone he knows should be with him at least for the initial sedation. Leave everything else to the vet. He will tell you what to do. The carcass will have to be collected. Here, too, you have a number of options, which the vet will be able to explain to you. Be somewhere else when the carcass is collected. There is nothing more you can do for your horse, and he no longer knows anything about it. Why fill your head with bad memories? It will also be easier for the person who collects the carcass, and will make his horrible job that much easier if he doesn't have to see you in floods of tears as well.

Unfortunately, for the sake of completeness, it was not possible to do without this chapter.

The last word

This is important. Amongst other reasons because my family, none of whom are horsey, always want copies of the book, and then only read the first and last pages before putting them on the shelf with the others ... Hello everyone, and bless you!

Then, of course, I have to take my leave of you, dear reader, and thank you for reading this far.

I hope that you will now be able to recognise an emergency and deal with it, and that you have learned the importance of preventive action. If something unforeseen does happen, you are now in a position to be able to handle and mitigate the situation competently.

Some chapters and descriptions may well come across as a little too light-hearted for the serious health problems they deal with. It is always deeply affecting to be faced with a sick horse, and feelings of sympathy are often accompanied by feelings of shame because people feel that they could have done more to prevent the accident, or at least make the situation better. The overriding thought is always for "the poor horse".

The jolly tone used in some parts of the book is in no way meant to convey that the subject should be taken lightly, but is an attempt to put the information across in an objective and readable way. Sympathy and sensitivity should never be lost in a welter of objectivity and blithe superiority. It is not intended that you should merely be able to help, but really, really want to help.

For your own and your horse's sake, I hope that you never have to help.